Take a Nap!
Change your life.

The Scientific Plan

To Make You Smarter,
Healthier, More Productive

Take a Nap!
Change your life.

Sara C. Mednick, Ph.D.

with Mark Ehrman

Workman Publishing • New York

Library of Congress Cataloging-in-Publication Data is available.

ISBN: 978-0-7611-4290-4

Workman books are available at special discounts when purchased in
bulk for premiums and sales promotions as well as for fund-raising or
educational use. Special editions or book excerpts can also be created
to specification. For details, contact the Special Sales Director at the
address below, or send an email to specialmarkets@workman.com.

Workman Publishing Co., Inc.
225 Varick Street
New York, NY 10014-4381
workman.com

WORKMAN is a registered trademark of Workman Publishing Co., Inc.

Printed in the United States of America
First printing December 2006

10 9 8 7 6 5 4 3 2 1

To our loving fathers—and the greatest
of nappers—Sarnoff A. Mednick and
(the late) Alexander Ehrman.

Acknowledgments

The authors acknowledge the scientists whose work provided the platform upon which this book now stands: in particular, *Power Sleep* author Dr. James B. Maas, who coined the term "power nap," Dr. David F. Dinges, who edited the first academic book on napping, and William C. Dement, M.D., Ph.D., "the father of sleep medicine," whose groundbreaking research imbued the scientific study of sleep with the respect and attention it enjoys today. We're also indebted to the work of the National Sleep Foundation and its tireless campaign to raise public awareness of the role of sleep in our overall health.

We furthermore want to thank everyone who lent a hand, an ear, an idea or a story in the making of this book, from conception to completion, particularly all the nappers and would-be nappers who shared pieces of their lives with us. Thanks also to everyone at PFD, especially our agent Zoë Pagnamenta, and to Peter Whybrow for steering us in her direction. And finally, this book would never have been possible without the positively inspiring staff at Workman—Paul Hanson, Peter Workman, Lynn Strong and Jen Pare, and especially our indefatigable editor, Susan Bolotin. You can all take a well-deserved nap.

Personally, I am grateful to the mentors who have encouraged me to place equal value on insight and intelligence and always to choose the path that leads to the greatest joy. In particular, I thank my mom and dad, Birgitte and Sarnoff Mednick, for their unconditional love and constant support; my brother, Thor, for never ceasing to inspire me; my sisters, Amy and Lisa, and their families for bringing music, poetry and beautiful babies to us all. Thanks to Bob Stickgold and Ken Nakayama and everyone at the Harvard Vision Lab and Sleep Lab for helping me learn to nap; Sean Drummond and Geoffrey Boynton and everyone at the Salk Institute and UCSD, for cocreating my new home in San Diego; and the National Institutes of Health, which generously supported my nap research over the years. Thanks to Bard College and my fellow die-hard individualists. To the best friends a person could wish for: Amriti, Roman, Meryl, Lilah, Karen, Hany, S.D.V., Kamala, Peter, Georgina, Laura, Colleen and Maureen, Mahshad and Constantine, and my beloved William. Finally, thank you, Mark Ehrman, for your elegant prose and friendship.

—S.M.

My own thanks goes out to my late father, Alexander, for always encouraging me to pursue writing even if he did believe that law school was the safer bet, and to my mother, Eva Deutsch, for all the love and support. A long-overdue appreciation to Sarah Jane Garretson for the doors you opened and for being my ally, confidante, counselor and comrade for all those years, and to my friends, T-Rik, John, Hunter, Jim and Theresa, Safini and Victor, Peggy, Lynn, Patricia, Burcu and Tulsa, who helped me through many less-than-heroic moments. Thanks to Charles Rappleye for the business lessons, Walter Gordon for the legal advice and the many editors over the years who've nurtured my career and taught me about the craft and business of writing—particularly Steve Randall (thanks for the lunches, too), Pamm Higgins, Mary Melton, Erik Torkells and Linda Friedman. Thanks to Sarnoff and Birgitte for periodically allowing your spectacular Hollywood Hills home ("Club Mednick") to be turned into a book-writing camp and, finally, to Sara for going on this journey with me.

—M.E.

Contents

Part Three: The Program

Introduction: The Couch at Harvard
My Journey from Skeptic to Nap Advocate

I t's 3 P.M. Wednesday. The phone is ringing. A student has dropped off a sheaf of printouts and expects me to make sense of them. I'm testing an experimental subject and the computer that's scoring the results has just crashed. In an hour, I'm scheduled to give a presentation of my research. What to do? After putting out the immediate fires, I have half an hour to spare. So I reach for my secret weapon. It never lets me down.

At 4 P.M., I enter the auditorium at the Salk Institute for Biological Studies, stand before my colleagues and explain my latest scientific findings on the benefits of napping. The presentation goes without a hitch. When I'm done, someone asks the question I get every single time I give this kind of talk.

"Do you nap?" he asks.

And I give my stock answer: "Of course I do. It's my secret weapon."

Five years ago, I never imagined that a healthy solution to facing life's multiple challenges could be as simple and attainable as a short nap. Faced with a challenge, I'd respond with another shot of espresso, splash some cold water on my face and drag myself through the rest of my day. If someone had told me that I would go on to become a "nap expert"—and a staunch advocate of the restorative powers of daytime rest—I would probably have advised psychological counseling.

But life-changing lessons come in all forms. In my case, the catalyst was a ratty old couch that arrived at my lab in Harvard University's Department of Psychology, where I was a graduate student. Its owner was about to throw it away (for good reason, by the looks of it), but Jay Edelman, one of the research associates, wanted something for visitors to sit on. I needled him endlessly as a trio of grad students carried that ugly brown couch into his office on the seventh floor of William James Hall. It probably looked fine the day it came home from the store, but after 20 years of duty its wool upholstery was pilling and cotton stuffing was curling out every-where. Little did I suspect that an old castaway couch would give me an education I couldn't get in any Ivy League lecture hall.

My preschool teachers can vouch for the fact that I was never much of a napper. Back then, teasing the boys and disrupting my fel-low students' rest seemed a much more interesting way to spend nap time. And until my encounter with that couch, not much had changed. But my father, also a research psychologist, swore by napping, and he wasn't the only accomplished person I respected who vouched for all the wonderful benefits a nap can bring. "Well, that's just their opinion," I thought. "Where's the proof?" My attitude was: "Time spent napping is time taken away from getting things done."

Of course, not all my great teachers were inanimate . . . or worn out at the seams. During my second year at Harvard, I walked into a lecture by Dr. Robert Stickgold, an associate professor of psychiatry. At that point, I had already burned through several possible thesis topics, tossing them all aside. I wanted to study something that would have a beneficial impact on a large segment of society, and investigating visual memory in schizophrenic patients—fascinating as that might be—didn't fit the bill. But it was immediately apparent that Dr. Stickgold's work was different.

He was investigating the role of sleep and its effect on different measures of learning and memory, such as how accurately subjects could tap out a specific sequence on a keyboard or how quickly they could pick out the orientation of lines that flashed briefly on a computer screen. While these tasks might appear pointless, they are functionally related to many essential behaviors. For example, doctors need these skills to quickly scan an X-ray for tumors, pianists use them to learn a piece of music, and secretaries and data-entry clerks depend on them every minute of their working day.

Dr. Stickgold's method involved testing his subjects twice on the same memory task, either with or without a period of nocturnal sleep between test sessions, then measuring the change in performance. Since he was monitoring electrical activity in the brain during sleep, he was also able to determine whether the quality of sleep affected the performance change. What he discovered was that only the subjects who slept through the night showed any improvement. He also proved that a minimum of six hours of sleep was needed for improvement to occur, and that subjects showed the most improvement when they'd had at least eight hours' sleep. This research struck me as important and relevant. After all, what could be more applicable to our daily existence than something we spend a third of our lives doing—or should be doing, anyway? I wanted in. But I didn't yet know where I would make my contribution.

During a meeting where graduate students were supposed to initiate possible research ideas, I made this offhand comment: "With all your results about the need for six to eight hours of sleep, isn't it ridiculous that so many people believe that a short nap has any benefits at all?"

"Well, my studies don't address naps," Dr. Stickgold replied. "I was looking at nocturnal sleep."

So off I went to the library to research everything that science had to say about the nap—what studies had been done, what the results suggested and what theories had been advanced to explain them. In other words, step one in any kind of scholarly inquiry.

After poring over academic journals and online databases, I realized how little nap research was out there. And what was available didn't address my question: Does a nap positively affect a person's ability to perform memory tasks? Sleep researchers had invented impressive-sounding jargon—"prophylactic napping" (in anticipation of sleep deprivation), "compensatory napping" (after sleep deprivation) and "operational napping" (on the job)— yet they hadn't proved that daytime sleep has beneficial effects on the general population. Most of the research focused on special populations such as long-haul truck drivers, graveyard-shift workers and military personnel. But what about the rest of us? There was nothing addressing the kind of people I knew who claimed they were benefiting from napping—well-rested, healthy people with regular sleep and work schedules. Did my dad and my friends have reason to be such staunch nap supporters, or had too much midday sleep simply gone to their heads? On this point, the scientific community had little to say.

I went back to Dr. Stickgold with a proposition. "Why don't we run your experiment again?" I asked. "Only this time, instead of having a night of sleep between testing sessions, the subjects would take a 60- or 90-minute nap during the day, or no nap at all." He agreed that this would be a worthy endeavor and signed on.

We were in for a big surprise. Both the 60- and 90-minute napping groups showed as much improvement as did the subjects who had had six to eight hours of nocturnal sleep in Dr. Stickgold's original experiment. On top of that, the non-nappers' performance deteriorated, meaning that without a nap their brains didn't work as well as they should!

So now I had demonstrated the power of the nap to be a scientific fact. But there was more to come. A scientific experiment needs rigorous safeguards against allowing our beliefs to affect the outcome, and this methodology often creates a disconnect between the facts we uncover and the way we lead our lives. In my case, the gap was particularly dramatic. I was a revved-up graduate student trapped on a hamster wheel of papers, exams, assisting faculty members and teaching undergraduate courses. Fifteen-hour days followed one after another, periodically expanding to 24-hour cycles without sleep. Before I could catch up, a bigger mountain of work would be dumped in my lap. I was losing focus, alertness and my ability to acquire and integrate information. My nerves were rattled from too much caffeine. I found myself getting irritated more often; sometimes, for the littlest things, I would burst into tears. Finally, one day, when even the ever-increasing shots of espresso could not keep my eyelids from fluttering shut, I crept into Jay's office and crashed out on his couch. Of course, I felt ashamed . . . and not just because I was always making fun of that old castaway. "This is a lab, not a Motel 6," I chastised myself. "Look at all the other grad students dutifully tapping away at their computers or running experiments. How would it look to be caught sleeping during the day?" I begged Jay not to tell anyone where I was.

Then one afternoon in my lab, as the numbers on the computer screen were dancing before my bleary eyes, I had my *Helloooo* moment: *Learning after a nap is equal to learning after a full night of sleep! Test scores of non-nappers deteriorate across the day!* That's what my research proved. Why should I feel guilty about napping when I was staring at evidence that it actually makes you smarter and more productive? I got up from my chair, turned to my lab partners and announced, "I'm going to take a nap."

I don't know whether giving myself permission to catch a bit of shut-eye made it easier for others to do the same, but pretty soon it was open napping season on the seventh floor of William James Hall. Brad, a lab partner who studied a fascinating syndrome called prosopagnosia (the inability to recognize individuals by their facial features), started taking a nap in the afternoon. Arni, our Icelandic import, would nap in the morning because he'd been up since dawn taking care of his newborn daughter. And Lorrella, who not only had a lovely three-year-old daughter at home but was pregnant with twins and drove all over the state of Massachusetts reaching her test subjects, took to napping whenever and wherever she could (including her car). My academic adviser, Ken Nakayama, took to napping in his comfortable leather chair with his feet on his desk. The only loser was Jay. With so much demand for his couch, we "voted" to move it into a room that could be darkened completely and started napping in shifts. I had created my first nap-friendly environment.

By then, it was clear to me that I would specialize in the long-ignored effects of napping. It had made me a more alert and productive person. Now the time had come to convince others that it could do the same for them.

And today, that's exactly what I do. My work at the Salk Institute has brought me into collaboration with the U.S. Navy, the Veterans Administration Medical Center, scholars at major universities, research organizations and private businesses. Many more scientists now recognize napping as a fruitful area of inquiry, and my endeavors in this field have been bolstered by the fine work of other individuals and institutions not only in the United States but around the world, particularly in Japan. A new branch of sleep research is establishing itself right before my eyes. While my early work investigated the effects of napping on learning, other people were studying its benefits on health, endurance and safety issues. Napping, as far as science is concerned, is finally getting some respect.

Still, many prejudices and misconceptions prevail. Ironically, the society that looks down its nose at napping is the same one that has been slowly robbing its people of more and more sleep. It's not as if the news hasn't gotten out. Media coverage has been very generous when new nap studies are published. Some innovative corporations and even whole towns have "woken up" to the benefits of napping. And I receive many e-mails from students who've brought couches or cots into their university studying areas, workers who nap at lunch and communities that have organized "napping clubs." But these developments are mere scattershot in the face of the major attitude adjustment that needs to take place.

That's why it was important to write this book.

The "big picture" message is that napping is a necessary and effective tool that can be used by anyone in pursuit of optimum health, happiness and productivity. I want to tell you why that is so, and how to make that knowledge work for you, your family, your company and your community. I want to make you a napper.

My cowriter and I bring more than a differing set of skills to the project; we also represent diametrically opposed lifestyles. My life is highly structured. I juggle my research at the Salk Institute with speaking engagements, conferences and correspondence. And, like everybody else, I have a personal life—relationships, social engagements, exercise and recreation. Yet I am certain that none of this would occur without penciling in a half-hour nap. Mark, on the other hand, is a freelance journalist who interviews prominent scientists and political figures when he's not reporting on travel destinations in Europe or the latest Hollywood gala. By necessity, he lives a largely unstructured life. Still, he organizes his workday around his naps.

The product of this napping collaboration is what you now hold in your hands. We hope you read it, believe it and put it to use.

Sara C. Mednick

Part One:
The Basics

CHAPTER 1

The new nap:

not your grandfather's siesta

I magine yourself in a perfect world. Your mood is positive. Your brain is operating at maximum efficiency. Your body feels healthy, energetic and agile. You have enough time to complete all the tasks at hand and still enjoy the company of family and friends. Every one of your goals is attainable.

In this wonderful land of your imagination, you enjoy a well-balanced diet, get enough exercise, breathe clean air and spend quality time with friends and family. What you *aren't* doing is walking around tired, right?

So ask yourself, "If I inhabited such a place, how much would I sleep?" Stumped? You're not alone. Most people don't get further than "a whole lot more than I'm sleeping now." After all, how do you remove the pressures of bills, job and relationships to create an oasis where you can even begin to envision what such a perfect world would involve?

Lucky for you, scientists have already resolved this issue. Our results back up what historians, anthropologists, artists and numerous brilliant leaders and thinkers have been telling their contemporaries throughout the ages. In a perfect world, all humans, including you, would nap.

It is written . . . in our DNA

L et's look at the rest of the animal kingdom. Do any other species try to get all their sleep in one long stretch? No. They're all multiphasic, meaning that they have many phases of sleep. *Homo sapiens* (our modern industrialized variety, anyway) stand alone in attempting to satisfy the need for sleep in one phase. And even that distinction is a relatively recent development. For most of our history, a rest during the day was considered as necessary a component of human existence as sleeping at night. As A. Roger Ekirch,

The witches of napping

Throughout early recorded history, working at midday was taboo in many cultures, since this was a time when otherworldly demons reigned—usually with a terrifying hand. The ancient Romans believed that nymphs cast evil spells of madness upon those who were out and about at midday, possibly because they observed that people who skipped their nap showed signs of mental disturbances. Evagrius of Pontus, a fourth-century monk, warned his fellow Christians about the spirit of *acedia*, who attacked during the midday hours and laid siege to the soul. Jewish rabbinic literature spoke of *iharire*, midday spirits who hovered just aboveground and threatened mayhem, while Arabic mythology believed the midday demon of Qeteb to be the worst of them all.

Perhaps the most colorful of these demons is Poludnica, whose name translates as "Lady Midday." Also known as Pszpolnica, this fearsome deity still roams the imagination of Slavic countries and is often pictured carrying shears, a symbol of death. In one version, she takes the shape of a young woman dressed in white who walks in patches of rye, grabbing the heads of those who work at noon and twisting their necks until they burn with pain. In another, she appears as a disheveled crone with a cane who captures children, bakes them and eats them for lunch—a specter invoked to frighten youngsters away from the family orchards while their parents nap. The fact that this terrifying apparition prowls the northern latitudes of Germany and Siberia underscores the notion that the warm Mediterranean cultures were not alone in their healthy horror of life without the nap.

one of the few historians to study sleep, put it, "Napping is a tool as old as time itself."

Does this mean that cave people napped? Well, little is known about sleep/wake habits back in the Stone Age, but the best guess is that sleep occurred throughout the day and night. Looking at contemporary primitive cultures, we find that the Gebusi of Papua New Guinea engage in multiphasic sleep. It makes sense that primitive peoples would sleep in short periods, since someone always has to keep watch for predators, but most of us no longer have to lose sleep over lions and tigers. With the advent of civilization, our sleep consolidated into fewer episodes, and eventually we fell into what scientists have come to realize is our fundamental, internally programmed pattern: biphasic sleep composed of one long period during the night and a short period in the middle of the day.

By the first century B.C., the Romans had divided their day into periods designated for specific activities, such as prayer, meals and rest. Midday became known as *sexta,* as in the sixth hour (noon by their way of counting), a time when everyone would go to bed. The word has survived in the familiar term *siesta.*

But hard scientific evidence that the nap is woven into our DNA didn't arrive until the modern era, when Dr. Jurgen Aschoff of the Max Planck Institute in Germany carried out a study that can only be described as peculiar. In the 1950s, Dr. Aschoff refurbished some abandoned World War II bunkers with all the amenities of small one-bedroom flats, except that they had no windows, clocks, televisions, radios or newspapers—no way to tell the date or time or even whether it was day or night. He then paid volunteers to live in them for a period of weeks, during which time he monitored their temperature, blood pressure and various other biological indicators. After a short transitional phase, subjects generally experienced one large dip in energy in the middle of the "night," when they would sleep six to seven hours; roughly 12 hours later, a mini-dip would drive them back to bed for a shorter period of sleep.

The post-lunch dip . . . without the lunch

Napper or not, you're no doubt familiar with that slump of energy that occurs just after lunch time. But is it actually what you've eaten—or how much—that makes you want to fall asleep the minute you leave the table? Or is it a function of your circadian rhythm? In study after study comparing sleepiness in subjects who had eaten lunch with those who hadn't, scientists have demonstrated that both groups are equally likely to feel drowsy in the early afternoon. Think about it: If it were the meal that made you tired, why wouldn't you feel like going back to bed after breakfast? Well, the morning is not when your programmed mini-dip occurs.

In other words, when people are forced to follow their own internal imperatives, the nap quickly reasserts its rightful place in the behavioral scheme. Subsequent studies proved this to be the case even among people who believed themselves incapable of napping, as well as in circumstances where they were specifically instructed *not* to nap!

The unseen hand guiding sleep and waking is our so-called biological clock or circadian (*circa* = around, *dia* = day) rhythm. This fundamental property of the human circuitry regulates sleep as well as body temperature, heart rate, growth hormone and urine production. But it doesn't just govern human biology. All living things—from a single blood cell to a two-ton elephant—dance to the beat tapped out by their circadian drum.

While Dr. Aschoff arrived at his discovery by accident, like a Christopher Columbus of human biology, University of Pennsylvania professor Dr. David Dinges was the first scientist to pose the direct question "Is napping natural?" In 1989 he brought together an impressive collection of sleep experts to examine napping across life span, occupation, culture and even species. A consensus emerged that not only is napping beneficial for alertness, mental ability and overall health, but our brains are actually programmed for it. "In examining sleep's orphan," Dr. Dinges concluded, "we found a lost progeny."

The siesta is dead. Long live the nap!

So how did we lose this progeny? We can start by blaming the clock. Between the 13th and 15th centuries, mechanical time-pieces replaced the sundial and water clock. The day, having previously been regarded as a series of experiences, could now be reduced to the passage of measurable units: seconds, minutes and hours. Workers began getting paid by the hour instead of by the job, and it didn't take long for the "Time is money" mantra to become the de facto law of the land. Sleep, especially during the day, began to be perceived as a waste of both. Interestingly, our English word *nap* traces back to the Old English word *hnappian*, "to doze," and first appeared in the 14th century.

As the Industrial Revolution progressed, biphasic sleep began to disappear from the more developed countries of northern Europe, particularly in the newly expanding cities. These cities were bursting with commerce, factories and culture, expanding the workload on individuals so that people were working longer hours and, unfortunately, at a younger age. The siesta survived in the less-developed south, because the intense heat of midday drove everyone—bosses and workers—to their beds. But eventually the march of progress reached the Mediterranean countries, and the siesta waned as they air-conditioned their environments and joined the competitive global economy. Today, only 7 percent of Spaniards living in big cities sleep during the day.

What's needed now is a program that will reclaim the nap without resurrecting the siesta, and here's where science must take the lead. Examining the habits of primitive tribesmen and ancient Romans won't help you create the time and place where you can restore your body to its natural rhythm if you're holding down two jobs and trying to raise a family. And while it's inspiring to know that Leonardo da Vinci, Isaac Newton, Napoleon Bonaparte and Albert Einstein refused to succumb to the madness of monophasic sleep,

citing their example probably won't convince your boss that napping at work will be good for your company's bottom line. You can
talk until you're blue in the face about the many U.S. presidents,
including John F. Kennedy, who believed in napping. You can cite
the example of Winston Churchill, who credited the nap with
winning the Battle of Britain: "We were not made by Nature to work,
or even to play, from eight o'clock in the morning till midnight," he
famously said. "We ought to break our days and our marches into
two." But none of these points will stem the anti-nap tide.

Scientists no longer argue about whether napping is natural or
unnatural, helpful or unhelpful. These are givens. We now explore
more technical questions, such as how duration, timing and quality
affect the benefits derived from a nap and how people outside the
experimental setting can reap those benefits on an everyday basis.
What we are doing is much more than simply identifying a human
behavioral trait. We are creating a new wellness technology.

Think of the Internet. Before people with vision realized the
potential of the World Wide Web, this network was a little-known
tool used primarily by specialized populations such as academia
and the Department of Defense. So, too, are emergent nap "technologies" poised to move from specialized subgroups to the population at large. NASA, for instance, devised a precise schedule of
in-flight naps that improved performance of pilots on extended
flights. Numerous airlines and railroads, including British Airways,
Air New Zealand and Amtrak, have adopted the program. Why
shouldn't these powerful tools be available to you?

In 2002–03, my colleagues at Harvard and I conducted a series
of studies looking at naps in normal populations. We proved not only
that a nap can restore proficiency in a variety of critical skills that
we rely upon every day, but also that certain kinds of naps can produce improvements previously observed only after a full night of
sleep. Even more groundbreaking was the discovery that we can
combine the specific stages of sleep to target areas of improvement

more precisely. In other words, we can create "designer naps" that allow students, mothers, the elderly and nine-to-fivers to tailor their own regimens to suit their individual needs. Using our knowledge of sleep's effects on the brain and body, naps can now be integrated into our lives in a more targeted, efficient manner.

As a result, we have entered a new napping age. We now know that it's not necessary to shutter an entire city during a regular siesta time to keep people healthy, alert and well rested. We also know that, with the help of science and a little attitude change on your part, you are now in position to bring a bit of that perfect world into your life today.

And not a moment too soon.

CHAPTER 2

Fatigue:

a hidden epidemic

J ust after midnight on March 24, 1989, the *Exxon Valdez,* a floating behemoth laden with 53 million gallons of crude oil, was sailing the dark, icy waters off the southern coast of Alaska. The ship's captain, Joe Hazelwood, had drunk more than his share of vodka and had retired to his cabin . . .

Filling in for the captain, Third Mate Gregory T. Cousins knew they were approaching Bligh Reef but failed to notice that the tanker was on autopilot and thus not responding to his call for a change in course. As a result, the reef sliced through the hull, spilling a fifth of the toxic cargo into Prince William Sound, wiping out 250,000 seabirds, 2,800 sea otters, 300 harbor seals, 250 bald eagles, 22 killer whales and billions of salmon and herring . . . and fouling 1,300 miles of heretofore pristine coastline.

What does a 10-million-gallon oil slick have to do with a nap? The National Transportation Safety Board investigation attributed the accident to the fact that Cousins, who had been awake for 18 hours prior to taking the helm of the *Valdez,* failed to "properly maneuver the vessel because of fatigue and excessive workload." Given what science can tell us about the deleterious effects of sleep deprivation on decision-making, alertness and coordination, a case can be made that had Cousins simply lain down for a brief sleep, one of the greatest environmental catastrophes in recent memory—and the $2.5 billion cost for cleanup—might have been averted.

While the fate of the *Exxon Valdez* represents perhaps the most dramatic reason for reintroducing the nap into our culture, it is far from the only one. The pace of life has accelerated to the point where all of us must ask if there is a *Valdez* waiting to happen in our lives.

The walking tired

I magine a silent epidemic wreaking havoc on our health, endangering our safety and straining our relationships with family and loved ones. The body count rises dramatically, yet no presidential task forces are assembled, no big celebrity fund-raisers are held and very little outcry is heard in the media. As a result, millions of afflicted people go on as if nothing is amiss and the spread of the disease continues unabated. This is no imaginary scenario. The plague is upon us. It's called fatigue.

For decades, with hardly anybody noticing, one of our most precious natural resources has been ebbing away. Sleep. What might be called the recommended daily allowance is eight hours, but who among us gets nearly that much? According to the latest statistics by the National Sleep Foundation, almost 50 million Americans suffer from sleep deprivation.

Working late has become the new norm. On average, Americans spend 46 hours per week at their place of employment, and 38 percent work more than 50 hours, while in Canada the National Work-Life Conflict Study of the Canadian Safety Council has found that hours on the job are increasing there, too. Only in South Korea are work hours longer than ours. According to a recent report in the *Chicago Tribune* (September 2005), 7.6 million of us hold two jobs simply to make ends meet. And we're commuting longer hours to get to those jobs. Something has to give. And most

11

often, we choose what we erroneously believe to be the most expendable commodity: sleep.

Before Thomas Edison's lightbulb, our great-grandparents would get as much as 10 hours' rest during an average weeknight. Today, we're lucky to get eight hours on the weekend. The amount of actual weeknight slumber has shrunk, on average, to an alarming 6.7 hours. We are a nation of the walking tired, so much so that 51 percent of the workforce reports that sleepiness on the job interferes with the volume of work they can do. One in five adults is so sleepy that it interferes with his or her daily activities a few days a week, while an additional 20 percent report impairment a few days a month.

Once the nation with the most productive workforce in the world, the United States, by a number of measures, has fallen behind countries such as France and Germany. Our standard of living is slipping. Our students are underperforming. Our collective health is deteriorating. In areas such as science and technology, we no longer dominate. Politicians, pundits and experts from all fields have made an industry out of explaining what's going wrong. But continually overlooked is the role of that quiet little demon: fatigue.

Asleep on the job: a threat to safety

Asleep-deprived population is a dangerous population. And no one, not even the most rested of us, is safe. While the *Exxon Valdez* may be the most egregious example of the dangerous ramifications of sleeplessness, fatigue has been cited as at least a contributing factor in many of the worst disasters in recent history—the Union Carbide chemical explosion that killed thousands of people in Bhopal, India, and the nuclear catastrophe at Chernobyl, to name just two.

Here's why: No single organ is affected by lack of sleep more than the brain. In order to function, it must metabolize the glucose that it receives via the circulation of blood. Neither process is possible without sleep. Positron-emission tomography (PET) and functional magnetic resonance imaging (fMRI) scans, specialized imaging technologies that show changes in brain metabolism related to mental processing, performed on sleep-deprived subjects reveal that blood flow is most compromised to the thalamus, prefrontal cortex and inferior parietal lobe. These three components of the brain play critical roles in decision-making, attention span and the speed at which we adapt to new information.

At the front

Even the most intensive physical training offers no exemption from the cruel calculus of sleep deprivation. Studies commissioned by the Department of Defense and the Defense Advanced Research Projects Agency found that lack of sleep degrades not only the ability of combat soldiers to identify and locate the enemy, but also—and even more disturbingly—their capacity to care whether they succeed or not. Think of how this bears on the escalating incidents of friendly fire. In World War II, for instance, 21 percent of U.S. casualties were the result of actions by Allied forces. In Vietnam, the figure rose to 39 percent. In the Gulf War, 45 percent of American casualties were attributed to friendly fire. And in the first week of the war in Iraq, that number rocketed to a staggering 66 percent. As retired Special Forces Major F. Andy Messing Jr., executive director of the National Defense Council Foundation, put it at the time, "The biggest killer is fatigue, and right now we have a whole army running toward Baghdad on zippo hours of sleep."

The military's solution is to dose our fighting men and women with stimulants to keep them going and "alert." The problem with this approach became abundantly clear in January 2003, when Air Force majors William Umbach and Harry Schmidt faced court-martial after a friendly fire incident over Kandahar, Afghanistan, that killed four Canadian soldiers and wounded eight others.

Umbach's counsel publicly revealed what had previously only been whispered in the halls of the Pentagon—that the pilots' judgment was impaired because superiors pressured them to take "go pills" containing the powerful amphetamine Dexedrine and, moreover, that the practice was widespread.

Those revelations hardly curbed the practice. The most common stimulant given to men and women in the armed services is Modafinil, a compound sold to the general public as Provigil. This compound delivers all the wakefulness of amphetamines but none of the euphoria and is therefore believed to have little recreational use. Originally offered to patients with Parkinson's, Alzheimer's and multiple sclerosis, it was subsequently approved by the FDA for such "conditions" as excessive daytime sleepiness, a fancy term for extreme tiredness. The brand has garnered $200 million in sales for its maker, Cephalon, and other companies are rushing similar products onto the market, not just for the military but also for the domestic army of the walking tired. But short-circuiting the urge to sleep doesn't remove the need to sleep. "No drug has yet been invented that is a substitute for sleep," says Dr. John A. Caldwell, principal research psychologist for the Warfighter Fatigue Countermeasures Program. The alternatives only foster a false sense of staving off the effects of fatigue, a condition I call Fatigue Denial.

Behind the wheel

Anyone who has ever tried to find an affordable house in Los Angeles will understand why a husband and father would choose to commute to his Hollywood job from Bakersfield, some 120 miles away. But while he's saving money, this long-distance driver is endangering his own life and putting others at risk. Every morning, he's up before dawn so he can make it over the mountains to his job by 9 A.M. In the evening, it's another long, dangerous drive, often in the dark and sometimes through rain, fog or snow. Although he hasn't had a serious accident, there have been too many close calls.

Maggie's Law

In October 2002, Representative Robert Andrews (D–NJ) introduced the first federal bill focusing on drowsy driving. The bill, titled HR 5534, included "incentives for states and communities to develop traffic safety programs to reduce crashes related to driver fatigue and sleep deprivation." Also included were provisions for police officer training, the creation of a driver's education curriculum, the standardized reporting of fatigue-related crashes on police report forms and the promotion of countermeasures such as continuous shoulder rumble strips and rest areas.

The bill, which passed in August 2003 and became law in January 2004, was named after Maggie McDonnell, a 20-year-old college student from Andrews' congressional district in New Jersey. McDonnell was killed by a drowsy driver on July 20, 1997.

This man's plight is far from unique, but his accident-free record is not the norm for sleep-deprived drivers. The National Transportation Safety Board attributes more than 100,000 highway crashes per year, causing 71,000 injuries and 1,500 deaths, at least in part to sleep deprivation. Factor in non-highway accidents and the death toll rises much higher. How comfortable can you be on the road knowing that more than half of American adults report that they've driven while drowsy, especially when you consider the studies showing that sleepiness decreases attention and alertness by 50 percent? Or how about the fact that nearly one in five drivers reports drifting off behind the wheel, with that figure climbing to nearly one in four among 18-to-29-year-olds?

"It's just as bad as having five drinks and getting in the car," says Mark Hammer, spokesperson for New York's Institute for Traffic Safety Management and Research. Studies have shown that motorists who get only six hours of sleep are more likely to cause a crash than are those with a blood alcohol level of 0.05. With each additional hour of sleep deprivation, we are ordering another cocktail. After 24 hours of sleep deprivation, the impairment is equivalent to a blood alcohol content of .10, which is well past the legal limit in every state. Also, these studies warn us that the effects increase with each additional night of insufficient sleep. If there were the equivalent of a blood alcohol test for the sleep-deprived, we would be taking keys away from many more drivers.

Warning: Losing sleep is hazardous to your health

When we sacrifice sleep, we not only endanger public safety, but we also hurt—and even kill—ourselves. After air, food and water, sleep is the most critical necessity for maintaining the body's vital organs and systems. While death from lack of sleep is possible, it's the cumulative health effects of chronic deprivation that should be setting off alarms.

Study after study has found that decreased levels of nocturnal sleep are associated with increased risk of breast cancer and colon cancer, as well as disregulation of hormones that control appetite. It's about time for our surgeon generals, who rightly warn us about the evils of cigarette smoking, to put a little effort into raising consciousness about the dangers of sleep loss. A study of 70,000 women showed that heart attacks increased in those who slept less than seven hours per night; those who slept five hours had a 40 percent higher rate of coronary artery disease or heart attack. If our population is going to pay so much attention to its cholesterol, shouldn't we also start to think about our sleep? Sleeplessness causes hypertension, which can also lead to strokes. This is because blood pressure decreases during sleep. So when you remain awake longer than normal, your blood pressure remains higher than normal. Our immune system suffers, too, since the number of natural killer cells created by our bodies to fight off invaders is reduced by sleep deprivation,

Lack of sleep will not make you slim

If you harbor the illusion that going long periods without sleep will at least keep you thin, forget it. Sleep-deprived people become more susceptible to obesity and, consequently, arteriosclerosis and diabetes. A University of Chicago study found that subjects restricted to six hours of sleep a night for as few as four nights already showed increases of insulin in the bloodstream similar to what happens in a prediabetic state. When we deprive ourselves of sleep, the brain sends a signal that we are entering a period of overdrive and need extra energy to support our mental and physical functions. This causes us to crave high-fat, high-glucose body fuel—in other words, junk food—another reason why Americans can be both the hardest workers on the planet and the most overweight.

And practitioners of the Zone, Atkins and South Beach diets take note: Inadequate sleep causes decreases in the hormone leptin, restricting the body's ability to break down carbohydrates.

leaving us vulnerable to colds and flu, allergies and asthma, and increasing our risk of many types of cancer. By lowering testosterone, sleep deprivation can cause sexual dysfunction (in both men and women). Moreover, because cell repair is enhanced by sleep, lack of sleep has been shown to cause premature aging.

The mental health picture is equally depressing. Studies have conclusively linked sleeplessness to irritability, anger, depression and mental exhaustion. This is not only because the brain is affected; other organs and body functions are, too. The thyroid gland, which plays an important hormonal role in emotional stability, is dependent on adequate sleep. Other disorders with psychological components, including migraines, ulcers and eczema, are exacerbated by chronic sleep deprivation. Ever wonder why so many hardworking commuters experience road rage? One reason is that their lack of sleep is literally driving them crazy!

If this picture of sleep deprivation is looking a lot like stress, it's no coincidence. In a clinical sense, the two are indistinguishable.

We take stress very seriously. We read books so we can learn about its causes and cures. We turn to yoga and meditation, and we pamper ourselves at spas. Fatigue, meanwhile, gets short shrift. The truth is, there's a good chance we're confusing the two. For instance, studies show that the number one cause of work-related stress is working more hours. And what's the net result of long hours? Less sleep. Many of the people we label "stressed out" are nothing of the sort. They simply need to go to bed.

Both sleep deprivation and stress result in elevated levels of the hormone cortisol. Synthesized in the adrenal cortex, cortisol helps to regulate our blood pressure, heart rhythm and ability to break down carbohydrates and fats. (It's referred to as a catabolic hormone, which means its function is to break things down.) The end product is increased glucose in the bloodstream, which leads to greater energy. In and of itself, this is not a bad thing. However, every biological process must exist in balance and harmony with its opposite. In the case of cortisol, this opposing force is growth hormone, which allows the body to repair tissue that has been raided to produce the needed glucose. Sleep deprivation decreases growth hormone, limiting the body's natural ability to make necessary repairs. This is where things take a sinister turn. Without the restorative balance made possible by sleep, cortisol becomes a corrosive killer.

The Type A Fallacy

So here we are, risking life, health and well-being. What are we gaining in return? Less than you might think. A lot less.

Many people fall for what I call the Type A Fallacy, the argument that the more you work, the more productive you will be. An estimated 45 percent of adults say they will sleep less in order to accomplish more. Certainly many businesses have adopted that ethic, since employers keep expanding the workweek well past the 40-hour mark. But does this strategy pay off? No, at least not in terms of efficiency, productivity or profit.

A 2003 report by Circadian Technologies, Inc., a leading international consulting firm specializing in extended work hours, states that a 10 percent increase in overtime in manufacturing operations results in a 2.4 percent decrease in productivity; in white-collar jobs, performance can decrease by as much as 25 percent when workers put in 60 or more hours per week for prolonged periods of time. The report also found that sleep deprivation leads to increased ergonomic injuries (e.g., carpal tunnel and other repetitive-movement syndromes), which in turn result in lost workdays and higher workmen's compensation claims. A Cornell University study found that tired workers cost U.S. industry $150 billion a year in reduced job productivity and fatigue-related accidents. To put it in the language of the bean counters, sleep deprivation damages the bottom line.

Nowhere is the fallacy of "work more/do better" more vividly on display than on our college campuses, where students routinely pull all-nighters. Here again, research (some of which emanates a stone's throw from those dorm rooms) demonstrates that this strategy leads to failure. A 1997 psychology/sleep study at Bradley University found that students who stayed awake all night believed they performed better the next day than their counterparts who had eight hours of sleep. As it turned out, these students were in for a rude surprise. Their scores were worse. A similar experiment demonstrated that even subjects with six hours of sleep showed performance deterioration with a similar overestimation of their performance. We're back again to Fatigue Denial. The overtired have little insight into the deterioration of their performance, much like the guy leaving the bar who mutters, "I'm okay to drive."

The youngest victims

It is no exaggeration to say that sleep deprivation starts in the cradle. We are passing fatigue off to our children like secondhand smoke.

A newborn baby should get 14 to 15 hours of sleep per day, but most get only around 12.8 hours. By elementary school, children

19

require 10 to 11 hours of sleep but average only 9.5 hours. Adolescents should be sleeping between 8.5 and 9 hours per night, but only 15 percent of teenagers actually get that much.

Hyper-parenting, the urge to overschedule the lives of our young sons and daughters, has been robbing children of much-needed sleep. "Rest period" and "nap time," once as much a part of childhood as arithmetic and home economics, have been disappearing at an earlier age. And as is the case with adults, the hoped-for net gain in "productivity" (if such a thing should even be associated with children) doesn't add up. A study of adolescents' daytime functioning found that students who regularly got Cs, Ds and Fs in school were sleeping significantly less than A and B students. Additionally, those with less than seven hours of sleep on weeknights reported depressed mood, sleep/wake behavioral problems and attention deficit disorder, along with a generally poorer academic performance.

Parents are driven equally crazy by their teenagers' "laziness" and by their inability to fall asleep at a reasonable hour and get up without a struggle. But guess what? It's not the kids' fault. Renowned adolescent sleep psychologist Mary Carskadon has shown that children moving into adolescence experience a shift in their internal clocks. Teenagers naturally go to sleep later and wake up later. But instead of compensating for this circadian shift, high schools start their days even earlier than elementary and middle schools, robbing kids 13 to 19 years old of an additional 40 to 50 minutes of sleep per day.

To make matters even worse, high school administrators across the country are filling the early morning classes with the most demanding courses, under the erroneous assumption that alertness will be highest when the students are "fresh." In fact, Carskadon, who used actigraphy watches to keep track of each subject's sleep/wake behavior, found that many students actually nodded off during their earliest classes.

A culture of ups and downs

Take a walk down any business street or mall, and you'll notice something that wasn't there 10 years ago: a Starbucks, or some other coffee chain outpost. There aren't many dots to connect between the skyrocketing sales of caffeine and the precipitous decline in sleep. Today, 8 in 10 Americans drink coffee, with an estimated 3 million new drinkers added each year. The amount each individual consumes is increasing by 6 percent a year (from 3.1 to 3.3 cups per day). In Silicon Valley, California, overworked dot-commers made a national brand out of Red Bull, a beverage consisting of sugar (another substance people reach for when they need quick energy) and 80 milligrams of caffeine. The market is so bullish that you can find caffeine not only in soda—often in Jolt! proportions—but also in bottled water and even chewing gum. Other stimulants, such as guarana, a common additive in energy drinks, and yerba mate tea have begun making inroads into the American market as well.

The irony here is that all this caffeine ingestion produces the very condition it's supposed to alleviate—a classic vicious cycle. In its pure form, caffeine is a bitter-tasting white crystalline powder. In the brain, it works by binding to adenosine receptors and preventing adenosine from doing its job, which is to make us feel drowsy. Used in moderation, caffeine is not a demon drug; it can be useful as a quick energy boost and it can increase alertness. The problem is that not only are the benefits fleeting, but they're only productive when its usage is limited. That immediate pick-me-up you feel is real, but so is the inevitable letdown. And as with all addictive substances, greater dependency leads to less effectiveness as the liver learns to filter the drug more effectively—a process known as tolerance. But rather than letting our bodies recover, we keep increasing our caffeine intake until we're chugging it down in supersize doses. This excessive use raises blood pressure and causes irregular heart rate, accelerated breathing, anxiety ("coffee jitters") and, worst of all, sleep disturbance.

And then, once we've ingested enough stimulants to stave off fatigue, what do we do when we need to wind down? Here again, the pharmaceutical industry steps in, this time with Ambien to help us sleep, Xanax to stave off anxiety and Viagra to perpetuate the sex lives of the otherwise exhausted. But all these drugs have side effects, the kind you hear rattled off at the end of drug commercials. In the case of Ambien, you have to watch out for daytime drowsiness, dizziness, lightheadedness, difficulty with coordination, memory loss, tolerance, dependence and changes in thinking and behavior. For Xanax, add irritability, agitation, mental confusion, sleep disturbance, lethargy, muscle spasm, weakness and changes in libido.

And that's not even taking into account the many people who choose to medicate themselves without a doctor's supervision. The road from stress and fatigue to the abuse of drugs and alcohol is well known and well traveled, a situation exacerbated by the tendency of those who go this route to eat less nutritious foods.

Okay, that's a grim picture, but what is there to do? We can't create a 25th hour, nor do the forces pushing people into longer workdays show any signs of abating. But recent breakthroughs in sleep research show that the simplest solution lies in restoring the nap, a resource as old as history itself.

CHAPTER 3

The nap manifesto:

what napping can do for you

I t's free, it's nontoxic and it has no dangerous side effects. Hard to believe, with these powerful selling points, that people have to be convinced to nap. But alas, for way too long, napping has been given a bad rap.

Employers want to keep their workers occupied with the business of business. Parents want their children to do homework when they come home from school or at least to play outside instead of "sleeping the day away." University administrators think the sight of students napping on campus sets a bad example. But as the facts pile up, the case for napping becomes too compelling to dismiss.

If you're a closet napper, come out and show some pride . . . help your fellow employees, family members and friends to see the light. And for those of you who still insist on saying, "Give me one good reason why I should nap," science can do better than that. It can give you 20 reasons. Napping will allow you to:

1. Increase your alertness. This is, for many, the most important benefit. Whether you're on the road, observing market trends, diagnosing patients or interacting with clients, staying alert is the most important determinant of your efficiency. NASA studies have conclusively demonstrated that alertness increases by as much as 100 percent after a brief nap, even in well-rested subjects.

2. Speed up your motor performance. While most people think of motor learning in terms of an ability to play guitar chords, improve a swim stroke or perform a plié, you don't have to be a musician, athlete or dancer to benefit from faster motor performance. All of us engage in tasks that involve coordination, whether we're typing at a keyboard, operating machinery, changing a tire or bagging groceries. A Harvard study demonstrated that the speed of a learned motor performance is the same in nappers as in those who have had a full night of sleep.

3. Improve your accuracy. Making mistakes costs time, money, energy and sometimes even people's lives. While greater speed usually involves sacrificing accuracy, napping offers a valuable exemption from this general rule. So whether you shoot baskets or firearms, play sonatas or golf, cut diamonds or hair, a nap helps you get it right.

4. Make better decisions. What are you going to eat for lunch? Should you ask for a raise or wait awhile? What stock should you buy? Or should you sell? Every day, all day, we make decisions—both trivial and huge. Of course, some decisions are so significant that lives can hang in the balance. Airplane takeoffs and landings require high-precision timing and the ability to read, monitor and react to a wide variety of controls. Pilots who are allowed to nap in the cockpit commit fewer judgment errors on takeoff and landings than those who aren't.

5. Improve your perception. Think how much you depend on your eyes, your ears and, to a lesser extent, your taste, touch and smell. Without the ability to fine-tune your sensory/perceptual systems, you wouldn't be able to hone in on the important environmental messages and filter out the mass of distracting sensory information that bombards all of us on a regular basis. Research shows that a nap can be as effective as a night of sleep in improvement of perceptual skills. Driving, cooking, appreciating music or art, reading, proofreading, quality control and even bird-watching are all enhanced after a nap.

6. Fatten your bottom line. Fatigue-related accidents cost U.S. industry over $150 million a year. Businesses that allow their employees to nap have shown decreases in errors and increases in productivity. According to the Shiftwork Practices survey issued in 2004 by Circadian Technologies, workmen's comp costs are highest where employees report the most fatigue, and claims at facilities that ban napping are four times higher than those that allow it. Judged by this standard, naps are a bargain.

7. Preserve your youthful looks. Nothing ages you like fatigue. Adding a nap to your regimen will improve skin and tissue regeneration and keeps you looking younger longer. Napping is truly beauty sleep.

8. Improve your sex life. Sleep deprivation dampens sex drive and sexual function. Napping reverses those effects. So nap now and your partner will love you more later.

9. Lose weight. Studies show that sleepy people reach for high-fat, sugar-rich foods more than people who are rested. Take a nap and not only can you resist those potato chips and cheesecake, but you'll be producing more growth hormone that reduces body fat.

10. Reduce your risk of heart attack and stroke. Studies conclusively show that fatigue contributes to hypertension, heart attack, stroke, arrhythmia and other cardiovascular disorders even in otherwise physically fit subjects. Add a nap to decrease your risk for all these maladies and live a longer, healthier life.

11. Reduce your risk of diabetes. Sleep deprivation increases insulin and cortisol levels, which can raise the risk for type 2 diabetes, the sixth leading cause of death in the United States. Napping after meals will build up your defense against diabetes while improving the way you process your sugars.

12. Improve your stamina. Whether you're running a marathon or simply sitting through a series of meetings, a well-planned nap will keep you from fading out before the finish line. Studies have shown that a nap during or after work allows you to be as alert and ready for the second part of your day as if it were a brand-new day. So if you need to finish a deadline project or simply want extra energy to interact more fruitfully with your friends and family after a long day at the office, take a nap first.

13. Elevate your mood. While sleep deprivation causes irritability, depression and anger, napping bathes your brain in serotonin, reversing those effects and creating a more positive outlook.

14. Boost your creativity. It's no wonder that history's great artists and inventors took naps. Napping allows your brain to create the loose associations necessary for creative insight and opens the way for a fresh burst of new ideas.

15. Reduce stress. Stress and anxiety are the result of cortisol being produced in the adrenal glands. By releasing the antidote, growth hormone, a nap can reduce that stress and anxiety and make you a calmer person. So don't worry, start napping.

16. Help your memory. Much of your memory consolidation cannot occur in any meaningful way without sleep. Everything from learning a new language to remembering the periodic table of elements can be improved by adding a short nap between study periods.

17. Reduce dependence on drugs/alcohol. Deprive yourself of needed sleep, and you're more likely to abuse not only caffeine but alcohol and other drugs. A recent study from Denmark showed that people who complain of exhaustion are more likely to abuse drugs. Saying yes to a nap will make you less likely to reach for stimulants to keep you awake and downers to get you to sleep.

18. Alleviate migraines, ulcers and other problems with psychological components. In one way or another, cortisol is involved in all these ailments. By reintroducing growth hormone, napping can reduce their severity. Many doctors actually recommend a cold compress and a nap to relieve migraines.

19. Improve the ease and quality of your nocturnal sleep. Sure, it sounds contradictory, but sleeping during the day helps you sleep better at night. "Overtired" isn't just a figure of speech. Going past the warning signs of fatigue can push you into a slightly manic state in which your body revs up so fast to compensate for lack of sleep that you can be too "wired" to fall asleep when you have the opportunity. Now doctors have begun recommending treatment of syndromes as severe as narcolepsy and excessive daytime sleepiness through a structured program of naps. So nap now and sleep better tonight.

And finally . . .

20. It feels good. Okay, there's no way for science to really measure this, but millions of nappers can't be wrong.

Part Two:
The Principles

CHAPTER 4

The stages of sleep:
building blocks of the nap

B efore diving into the new nap technology, let's talk about sleep in general. From a clinical perspective, the components of sleep are the same whether they occur at 1 A.M. as part of an eight-hour stretch or in the middle of a 20-minute afternoon snooze. By taking this guided tour, you'll understand how the process works and how each element makes a unique contribution to overall wellness.

Okay, it's 11 P.M. You're in bed and drifting off into that mysterious realm. What happens now?

Well, lots, although science has only recently come to appreciate this. In ancient Greece, otherwise great thinkers such as Plato and the physician Galen espoused the idea that sleep originated from stomach vapors that rose up to the brain during digestion, cutting it off from the rest of the body and causing unconsciousness. Though theories would become far less convoluted over the ages, the notion of sleep as simply a shutting down of our physical and mental systems prevailed. In 1834, the Scottish physician Robert MacNish confidently declared, "Sleep is the intermediate state between wakefulness and death." How wrong this idea proved to be!

Waves and scans: the sleeping brain revealed

The evidence that changed medical definitions of sleep didn't arrive until 1929, when Johannes Berger devised an ingenious method to peek into the invisible workings of the brain. Attaching primitive electrodes to a subject's skull, he recorded electrical impulses from the brain on an apparatus that he called an electroencephalograph (EEG). In this manner, he was able to isolate different types of brain waves and observe that they were emitted during different mental states, such as falling asleep and being startled awake. All this was big news at a time when science could only guess what goes on inside the human brain. In 1937, through the use of the EEG, Wall Street tycoon, attorney and maverick scientist Alfred Loomis and his collaborators E. Newton Harvey and Garret Hobart identified five different stages of sleep, which they labeled simply A through E. Back then, these findings were regarded as a curiosity, and no one seemed to pick up on their significance until decades later.

The most famous discovery in sleep science occurred in 1953, when University of Chicago physiology professor Nathaniel Kleitman and Eugene Aserinsky stumbled on a phenomenon that would revolutionize our understanding of how people sleep. During an experiment, they observed that the eyeballs of sleeping infants darted left and right in sporadic bursts, coupled with irregular breathing and increased heart rate. Adults, they subsequently found, did this, too. They called this strange phenomenon rapid eye movement, or REM. What made this more than an "Oh, isn't that interesting?" piece of trivia was the fact that subjects reported vivid dreaming only during this period. This established once and for all that not only is sleep more than just the absence of waking—it isn't even correct to speak of it as a single, undifferentiated unit.

The most explosive breakthroughs occurred during the 1990s, when new technologies allowed neural operations to be analyzed down to the minutest molecular and genetic mechanisms. Science now had clear, instantaneous snapshots of "the angry brain," "the depressed brain" and even what a brain looks like (at least in terms of its metabolic or electromagnetic activity) when it's recalling a telephone number. In much the same way that quantum physicists have delved far beyond atoms and molecules and now study the behavior of quarks and neutrinos, sleep research was no longer limited to the effects of sleep in general. Instead, sleep was divided into five distinct phases—now known as Stage 1, Stage 2, Stage 3, Stage 4 and REM—and researchers systematically began mapping all the physical, chemical and biological characteristics of each one.

The sleep cycle

During sleep, the electrical activity in the brain taps out a catchy but unwavering rhythm that goes 1, 2, 3, 4, 2, REM, 2, 3, 4, 2, REM, 2, 3, 4, 2, REM . . . and so on. Each sequence is known as a "sleep cycle." Stage 1 occurs only once—as a transition into the sleep state. We spend over half of our total sleep time in Stage 2, about 20 percent in REM and the remaining time in Stages 3 and 4. An entire cycle lasts 90 to 100 minutes, about the length of the average movie.

So what dramas are enacted during each of these distinct events? Let's start that movie and find out.

Stage 1

As you sink into your pillow and close your eyes, a medium-frequency, medium-amplitude brain wave called alpha predominates as the beta wave diminishes. Your eyes roll slowly from left to right, and as you drift from relatively structured thought—reflecting on a discussion you had with your boss or contemplating the purchase

What's in a wave?

Brain waves are an expression of the two critical features of electrical activity: amplitude and frequency. Amplitude refers to the amount of energy discharged, i.e., how much of a jolt it packs, while frequency describes the number of discharges per second. By plotting these two values on a moving graph, we actually "see" these waves, much the same way that heartbeats are visible on an electrocardiogram.

WAVE

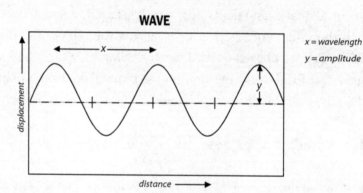

$x = wavelength$
$y = amplitude$

displacement

distance ⟶

This is important because different systems of the brain emit different charges, so that each can be represented by its own signature wave. Many are identified by a Greek letter—alpha, beta, delta, theta—while others get fanciful English names like spindles and "k" complexes.

By observing how the occurrence of these forms varies under specific conditions, we gain insight into how the brain behaves under a variety of physical and emotional states. The identification of the alpha wave and its association with relaxation, for instance, led to biofeedback techniques that produce the same calm brain signature observed in experienced practitioners of meditation.

of new tires for your car—your mental associations begin to loosen. Tires become rubber, rubber floats on the ocean, oceans have barges. Barge. Barge in. Barge into a room. Space. Floating in outer space . . .

As you cross the threshold of sleep into Stage 1, alpha subsides and generalized involuntary muscle contractions occur, accompanied by surreal visual imagery such as falling off a sidewalk. You may also find yourself momentarily paralyzed. It is possible to wake up during this period and have a terrible sensation of not having control of your body but being fully awake. Don't panic. It passes quickly.

Stage 1 lasts two to five minutes and is the least understood of all the components of sleep. It appears to be a quasi-REM state, involving nonlinear thoughts and associations, but it lacks REM's trademark eye movements. The technical term for this state is sleep-onset dreaming, although it has developed a rich lore under the heading "hypnogogic state." Actively cultivated by mystics, artists and mavericks who tout its wondrous effects, this oddity of sleep has yet to give up any of its secrets to science. As far as research can ascertain, it appears to be a warm-up exercise to prepare the mind and body for entry into the sleep state. We will return to the hypnogogic state in Chapter 9, but for now, let's move on to Stage 2, where the more charted territory of benefits begins.

Stage 2

After about two to five minutes, your heart rate slows and your body temperature drops. Without noticing, you've slipped into Stage 2 and true unconsciousness.

If sleep is a soup, then Stage 2 is its stock. Not only does it provide the medium in which all the other stages "float," but it's pretty nutritious all by itself. At the end of the 20th century, Stage 2 was still thought of as a transition phase between the so-called "real" stages of sleep (something to keep in mind before completely writing off Stage 1); today, the latest word from university laboratories is that our generous allowance of Stage 2 plays a dominant role in increasing alertness, one of the most critical benefits of sleep. The ability to grasp the significance of what our senses perceive is associated with the thalamus, which forwards our raw sensations to the proper brain areas for processing. No surprise, then, that this plum-size relay operator is taking its own nap during this stage.

Other areas of the brain begin to take it easy, too. These include the brain stem, the ball of tissue that sits atop the spinal cord and controls breathing, heart rate, reflex response and the neuro-motor aspects of speech; the prefrontal cortex, an area involved in language, abstract reasoning, planning, problem solving and social interactions; and the cingulate cortex, located just above the brain stem, which helps you override certain automatic responses for newly learned ones. The phrase "give your mind a rest" literally applies to these areas while they conserve energy not only during this stage, but even more so as the sleep cycle progresses.

The defining wave characteristics of Stage 2 are spindles and "k" complexes. Spindles are lightning-quick oscillations that increase and decrease in amplitude—all in under a second. On an EEG print-out, they appear to have tapering tails like the spindles used in spin-ning yarn. To understand what these electrical signals have to do with learning, think about the billions of neurons balled up inside

THE ELECTRICAL SIGNATURES

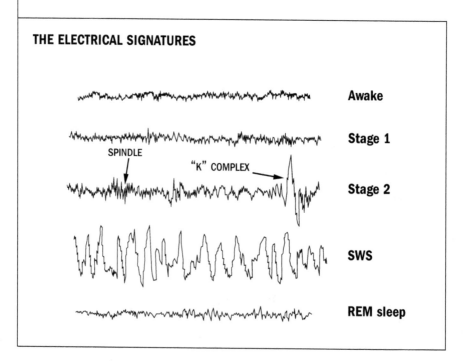

Awake

Stage 1

SPINDLE

"K" COMPLEX

Stage 2

SWS

REM sleep

your head. These nerve cells communicate with each other via chemicals called neurotransmitters. The release of a neurotransmitter from the tail of one neuron unlocks the receptor at the head of another, which in turn fires off an electrical signal to still another, creating a chain of chemically and electrically linked neurons. But since a neuron can be excited by any one of approximately 1,000 of its neighbors, some synaptic pathways between neurons must be more strongly established than others. This is why the more times you dial a phone number, the more likely it is that you'll remember it the next time. And why the more often you go horseback riding, the better rider you become. While the layman might be content with the adage "Practice makes perfect," a neuroscientist prefers to express this as "Neurons that fire together, wire together." The soldering of individual circuits out of a maze composed of billions of random brain cells is accomplished by a process known as potentiation. With each repetition of information or series of behaviors, the synaptic pathway becomes more defined. High-intensity neural firing produces even more durable bonds, a process called long-term potentiation, or LTP.

This is not to say that LTP cannot occur without sleep. Anyone can remember an address simply by constantly repeating it. If you travel enough times during a single day to a new location, you can learn the route before you ever go to sleep. And while motor learning gets a big boost from Stage 2, there are many types of learning that are greatly sped up or facilitated by other stages of sleep. In some cases, like the ability to quickly identify a visual form (think of how soldiers in World War II antiaircraft battalions had to rapidly distinguish the silhouettes of friendly planes vs. those of enemy bombers), learning skills will actually deteriorate without sleep.

Sleep spindles are the electrical signature of LTP in the motor learning network. They can be compared to the flash of the welder's torch, each spark indicating the creation of a more efficient grid. The result for us is that we can move with greater grace, skill, speed and coordination. While spindles can occur throughout the night, Stage 2 is a veritable spindle harvest and thus key to consolidation of motor learning; without it, our ability to learn the sequence of muscle movements in activities such as dancing, typing or driving, to say nothing of executing them with skill, would be severely impaired. Spindles also play a role in implicit learning, or the learning you do without realizing it, such as familiarizing yourself with a new neighborhood. Increased spindle production has also been correlated with higher scores on some IQ tests.

While we know that spindles occur only during sleep, what isn't clear is why some things are more easily learned without sleep while for others sleep is almost essential. The best guess is that simple things tend to be more easily learned without sleep, but getting many complicated components to gel requires a sleep episode. For example, when learning to ride a bike, you need to coordinate your musculature with your posture, balance, visual information and spatial direction in order to propel yourself properly on this moving object. Sleep can help you make all those connections, whereas without sleep you will just grow tired and usually do worse before you do better.

"K" complexes are large-amplitude spikes, with a slight dip at the end as seen in a cursive letter "k." They shoot out from the cerebral cortex, an area associated with all higher-brain functions. These characters venture out only in Stage 2, appearing once every 2 to 8 minutes and lasting up to 30 seconds each time.

The function of "k" complexes is still wrapped in mystery. Science's best detective work has determined that they're associated with changes in blood pressure and seem to be indicative of the brain's descent into slower wave activity—the sound, perhaps, of the switch being thrown to send you into deeper sleep. This slowing down of vital signs and brain wave activity will continue throughout the rest of the cycle.

Stage 3 + Stage 4 = slow-wave sleep

As you drift farther down the river of sleep, the temperature inside your head cools and the blood vessels constrict. An EEG will pick up the signal of the extremely slow delta wave, along with remnants of faster-frequency waves lingering from Stage 2. As you cross the threshold into Stage 3, you enter a deep, dark world known as slow-wave sleep, or SWS.

Low-key coughing and humming—noises that would wake you up during Stage 2—now go unheard. It will take a loud bang or a sound of particular relevance, like your name or the cry of your baby (but, oddly, not the cry of a stranger's child), to bring you back to the waking world. For children, the noise level can actually reach over 120 decibels (think jet plane or rock concert) before they abandon the cozy comfort of slow-wave sleep.

Your breathing is regular and stable, but noticeably shallower. The muscles responsible for holding the air passages open are less active, so you experience a 15 to 20 percent decrease in oxygen intake.

Checking your hormones now, we find that the cortisol spigot has completely shut off. This so-called "stress hormone" is no longer stripping away at your body tissue, wreaking catabolic havoc. Not only that, but the pituitary gland is spewing extra growth hormone to fix the damage. Besides promoting bone and muscle growth and protein synthesis, this hormone helps you metabolize fats (particularly cholesterol) and carbohydrates, processing them out of your body instead of adding to the supply on your hips or belly. ("Slimming while you sleep" is more than just a fantasy during slow-wave sleep!) During puberty, growth hormone is key to the development of sexual organs and muscles and bones. Prolactin, too, increases in the bloodstream, working to stimulate mammary gland development and milk production in new mothers.

During SWS, all the critical physical benefits of sleep are delivered. Like your own internal handyman, it restores your tissue and organs to peak condition, prolonging health and youthfulness while at the same time decreasing stress, anxiety and susceptibility to illness. No wonder you can sleep so soundly.

While your body undergoes this ambitious reconstruction project, the firing rate of your neurons drops to a sputter and your thinking brain can't seem to create more than the most rudimentary associations. Should someone wake you during SWS and ask for the first word that comes to your mind when you hear "doctor," you might answer "nurse," whereas during a stage more closely associated with creativity and dreaming, you might find yourself coming up with something further afield like "white" (doctor > nurse, nurse > white). And asked what you were dreaming about when you're roused from SWS, you'll likely respond with something as ordinary as taking out the garbage, whereas during REM, the classic dream phase, an elephant would have been taking out the garbage with you inside the trash can, and the elephant was your brother, and for some reason that was perfectly understood . . .

Does this mean that all higher brain functions switch to idle? No, because only under these low-wattage conditions do we meet long-term potentiation's opposite: a cool character known as long-term depression (LTD), whose signature tune is the low hum of the delta wave. During waking life, you accumulate a multiplicity of information and learned responses, each of which has forged its own synaptic pathway; this information can clog your neural communication network, making it more difficult for new learning pathways to form. LTD dismantles responses to memories that are no longer necessary by uncoupling the neural connections upon which they're based. This means that your tree of knowledge, pruned of its deadwood, grows bigger and stronger. Thus slow-wave sleep is not just the "heal your body" state for which it gets the most credit; it's also the most effective at clearing your mind. As an added bonus,

SWS has proven vital to the formation of declarative memory—new information consciously learned, such as a friend's birthday, a phone number or the periodic table of elements.

While it's tempting to regard Stage 4 as more of the same, we need to attune ourselves to a few subtle differences. The slowing of physiological processes continues, but what is unique here is the complete absence of the short, fast waves that were introduced in Stage 2. Stage 4 is our deepest sleep stage, and our systems show the greatest degree of downshifting from the waking state.

REM sleep

After a seven- or eight-minute rebound back into Stage 2, the most exciting stage begins. Irregular gulps of air replace the steady breathing of slow-wave sleep. Your heart rate speeds up, your blood vessels dilate and your blood pressure rises by as much as 40 percent. While your body temperature falls, a torrent of blood—50 percent above waking level—raises the temperature in your brain. The firing rate of neurons increases to its highest level, producing the beta wave that is characteristic of awake and active people. Your muscles twitch involuntarily while you simultaneously experience full-body paralysis. And, most characteristically, your eyeballs dart from side to side. Cue fanfare: REM has arrived.

Now you experience those vivid dreams that many of us find so captivating. This likely explains the paralysis—a built-in safeguard to prevent dreamers from actually acting upon their experiences. People in whom this mechanism fails have been known to leap out of bed and injure themselves as they flee wild beasts or a runaway freight train.

The human body does not regulate its temperature in REM. We don't shiver if the thermostat is turned down. Nor do we sweat if the heat is turned up. This is our most reptilian state—body temperature rising and falling in accord with that of the ambient environment. Should the thermometer rise or fall more than 10 degrees, such a state becomes unhealthy and the REM circus will fold its tents and leave.

Because the brain's electrical activity matches patterns observed during our waking hours, REM used to be called "paradoxical sleep." The alpha wave reappears along with beta, which is related to increased mental concentration. Truly a cacophony. But this is more like the controlled noisiness of a factory than the chaos of a battlefield. And how apt, since so much is being "manufactured" here.

The strange ways of REM sleep have made it the darling of sleep researchers. In their shower of attention, they have recently discovered heretofore unknown brain waves that they call PGOs, standing for the *p*ons, *g*eniculate nuclei (of the thalamus) and *o*ccipital cortex, where these waves are generated. Showing themselves in short bursts lasting roughly a tenth of a second, PGOs appear to produce potentiation—the welding of the brain's learning network. Furthermore, studies in animals have demonstrated a link between the appearance of these waves and memory improvement.

Also presenting itself in all its glory is science's newest fascination, the theta wave. Emanating at three to seven cycles per second from the hippocampus, theta appears to support information transfer between short-term memory "holding tanks" to areas of the brain where more permanent long-term memory storage occurs.

With all this memory-enhancing activity going on, it's no wonder that memory researchers speak of the "REM window" being opened. Without this critical period of sleep in the minutes to hours after a learning experience, no significant consolidation of that information will occur. Say you've spent the day going over complex grammatical structures of the Chinese language for a class, or the legal precedents for a case you're going to argue in court. You have only a short period to digest them, or they'll be wiped clean from your memory banks. Actors memorizing pages and pages of dramatic text will tell you that going to sleep right after studying their lines helps their retention. This strategy makes scientific sense because quickly going to sleep prevents any interference by competing information. More importantly, REM will change the weak neuronal connections that hold information to stronger bonds through added memory processing "offline." Unlike the more physical motor learning that results from Stage 2 spindles, the long-term potentiation of our higher-learning functions has to wait for REM.

Spatial orientation, the way you learn to navigate a new neighborhood or the virtual environment of a video game, needs REM if the results are to set in. Perceptual skills such as training your ear to hear important and relevant sounds—something a nighttime security guard would need to do his job effectively, for instance—don't get sharpened until this point in the cycle. Likewise, those who depend on visual learning—a bird-watcher who learns to spot different birds, a radiologist who must pick telltale patterns out of a monochromatic X-ray or a driver who must know how to spot hazards out his windshield—would have trouble executing these tasks if they were REM-deprived. Mastering anything complex, whether it be a mathematical formula, riding a bicycle or even reaching for a

A comfort zone

REM also plays a role in emotional memories. These are the associations we form between stimuli and emotions—the jingle of an ice-cream truck evoking the pleasure of eating a chocolate sundae, for instance, or the smell of a dentist's office reminding you of a painful root canal. REM solidifies the positive emotional memories while helping to uncouple associations that are no longer productive. This new discovery can play a supporting role in alleviating syndromes like post-traumatic stress disorder, whose victims exhibit exaggerated responses to stimuli that were once associated with some dangerous or traumatic event but are now innocuous.

And here's another plus: Studies have shown that people deprived of REM have excessive sensitivity to physical pain. Apparently your doctor wasn't just brushing you off when he promised you would feel better in the morning!

deeply creative solution, requires REM sleep to fuse these loose pieces of string needed to connect seemingly remote brain areas.

You can see that the popular notion of REM as simply a time for dreaming sells this crucial stage very short. Most of the activities that require higher brain processes—memory, creativity, complex learning—depend on REM to do their business.

To be continued . . .

You've just completed the first cycle of sleep. More than likely, after the REM show concluded you would remain asleep and return to Stage 2 to begin the cycle (minus Stage 1) over and over again until you wake up. Over the course of the night, you might pass through four cycles if you're getting enough sleep. But are all these sleep cycles identical? Even though the progression of stages never varies, is the time you spend in any given stage the same in every cycle? While Stage 2 can reliably be said to compose 60 percent of any given cycle, the other stages shift considerably from cycle to cycle. Understanding the mechanism that drives this proportionality, and how best to take advantage of it, won't affect the quality of your nocturnal sleep, but strange as it may sound, it's key to optimizing your personal nap. The reason for this lies in the fact that the story of sleep never ends. Morning comes, the alarm sounds, you make your coffee and head off to work, but something you thought you left on your pillow is actually following you.

CHAPTER 5

Dissecting sleep:

making a nap work for you

W hen you wake up from a good night's sleep, you haven't simply come out of a dark void; you've treated your body and mind to a sumptuous buffet whose three main dishes were Stage 2, SWS and REM. Much the same way that carbohydrates, protein and fat function in our diet, these three components form the basis of our sleep "nutrition."

And just as marathon runners carbo-load before a big race, weight lifters stock up on protein and heart patients benefit from increasing their intake of omega-6 fatty acids, we can adjust our sleep cycles to meet our individual needs. But here's the rub: During nocturnal sleep, our trip through Stage 2, SWS and REM is preprogrammed and we're just along for the ride. Only during a nap does the potential exist to cherry-pick stages based on the benefits we're looking for. So, on the day of that marathon, you might want a nap containing more Stage 2 for the motor enhancement that will keep your legs pumping, plus SWS to ease your pre-race jitters. But if you're going to French class, you may prefer extra REM to help you understand the complex structure of a foreign language.

All you need to do is calculate when a nap should contain an extra dose of any of these components and plan your nap time

That fuzzy feeling

Are you afraid of feeling groggy after a nap? Some people do, and what they're experiencing is sleep inertia. The culprit here is slow-wave sleep, not the nap itself. When you're fully awake, your brain is operating on many frequencies. But during SWS your entire brain rhythm has synchronized into a slow, uniform pattern. Sleep inertia is how we experience the lag that occurs while the brain once again re-creates the multiple faster frequencies. The groggy feeling can become particularly acute for the sleep-deprived, since someone whose body has a greater need of SWS has a greater chance of waking up during SWS and thus into sleep inertia.

The good news is that sleep inertia can be minimized by shortening or lengthening your nap to avoid waking up in SWS. You can also quickly "fire up" your brain through physical activity, sensory stimulation such as splashing water on your face or, if you must, having a shot of caffeine—all of which have been scientifically proven effective.

In any case, having napped cannot make you "more tired," any more than a light snack makes a starving person "more hungry." If you experience sleep inertia, you've simply whetted your body's appetite for a resource that your conscious mind has been trying to ignore.

accordingly. But how is such a thing possible? Remember the cliffhanger at the end of the previous chapter? When the story left off, you were well into your waking day but you were being tailed. And that mysterious presence was none other than the stages of sleep.

The shadow cycles

No biological process is an island. And sleep cycles do not end just because you've woken up. They continue as "shadow sleep cycles" across the day. As ghostly as this sounds, these cycles are governed by two reliably scientific principles: sleep pressure, which affects SWS, and circadian rhythm, which dictates the distribution of REM. Once you learn how these components behave, the benefits of your nap are at your beck and call.

Sleep pressure

From the moment you wake up, your body slowly builds the urge to go back to sleep. This phenomenon, born out of an increasing need for slow-wave sleep, is known as sleep pressure. In the morning, when your brain is relatively well rested, shadow sleep cycles will contain a small percentage of SWS. Later in the day, as the distance from your last sleep episode becomes greater, the amount of SWS also increases. Our brains have a homeostatic drive that always endeavors to maintain a balance between SWS and waking. Indeed, the generalized feeling of true sleepiness (the kind that is not related to being bored or physically overexerted) is simply the manifestation of our body's desire for SWS. If you stay awake indefinitely, sleep pressure intensifies until finally the urge to sleep overcomes any conscious resistance and you're "asleep at the wheel," or wherever you may be. SWS is a very demanding mistress. Her needs are not to be trifled with.

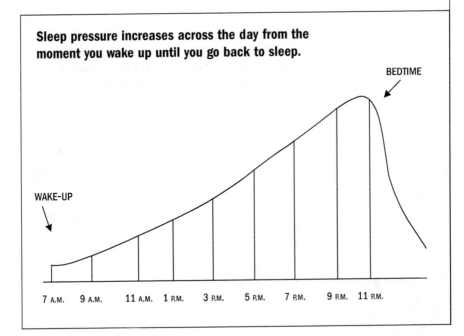

Sleep pressure increases across the day from the moment you wake up until you go back to sleep.

BEDTIME

WAKE-UP

7 A.M.   9 A.M.   11 A.M.   1 P.M.   3 P.M.   5 P.M.   7 P.M.   9 P.M.   11 P.M.

Once you do give in, the pressure drops with every passing cycle, much like air being allowed to intermittently escape from a balloon, so the earlier the cycle is within the nocturnal sequence, the more SWS it's going to contain. Later in your sleep, closer to morning wake time, sleep pressure has pretty much dissipated and the percentage of SWS in your last sleep cycle is relatively low. Likewise, naps across the day will vary predictably in terms of how much SWS they contain.

REM around the clock

Because slow-wave sleep is driven by sleep pressure, its rise and fall is contingent on an individual's sleep behavior. But REM sleep is a lot like the tide. It ebbs and flows, independent of human control. And just as the tide can be predicted by the phase of the moon, our propensity for REM, which is a function of our circadian rhythm, can be determined by simply looking at the clock. Sleep cycles generally contain the lowest amount of REM at 9 P.M., with the per-

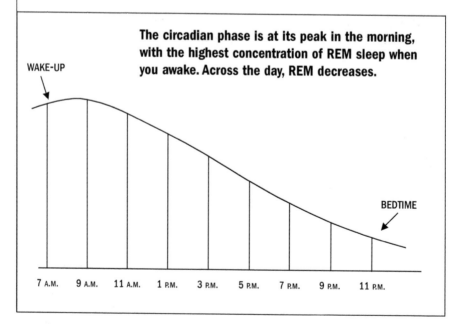

The circadian phase is at its peak in the morning, with the highest concentration of REM sleep when you awake. Across the day, REM decreases.

WAKE-UP

BEDTIME

7 A.M. 9 A.M. 11 A.M. 1 P.M. 3 P.M. 5 P.M. 7 P.M. 9 P.M. 11 P.M.

centage steadily increasing until 9 A.M. It then falls off again until it reaches its 9 P.M. trough, before beginning its inevitable climb all over again.

In people with normal sleep/wake cycles, REM and SWS pirouette nicely across the day and night. SWS predominates in the late afternoon and evening, when REM is in its natural low phase. Then, as we move toward morning and a higher REM cycle, sleep pressure has been relieved, so SWS doesn't hog the stage.

Your circadian rhythm also affects your body's energy level, temperature and many other biological functions. That's why you might feel like falling asleep at your desk at 3 P.M. but feel fine at a

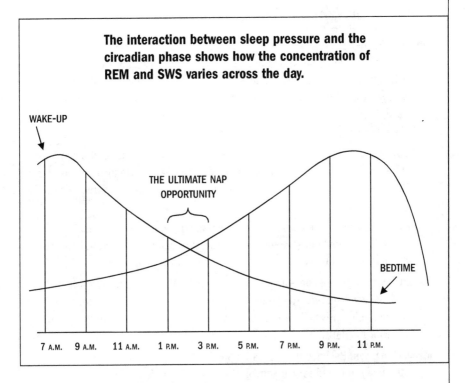

The interaction between sleep pressure and the circadian phase shows how the concentration of REM and SWS varies across the day.

WAKE-UP

THE ULTIMATE NAP OPPORTUNITY

BEDTIME

7 A.M. 9 A.M. 11 A.M. 1 P.M. 3 P.M. 5 P.M. 7 P.M. 9 P.M. 11 P.M.

post-work mixer, even though your sleep pressure has been rising steadily. Yes, your circadian rhythm brings you a "second wind," but you still haven't assuaged your need for slow-wave sleep. That accounting is still due.

Stage 2: the constant companion

Not much has been said about Stage 2 here. That's because it's the only constant in our equation. As the transitional element between all the major phases of sleep, Stage 2 comes between Stage 1 and SWS, between SWS and REM, and again between REM and SWS. No phase of sleep can be accessed without first passing through this important and beneficial portal. What is most important to remember is that the first time we enter Stage 2 in a cycle is

---

A Profile in Napping: **The law student**

Situation: Rasheed is a 22-year-old law school student who works two nights and one weekend day at a ladies' shoe store in a busy mall. He wakes up at 6:45 A.M. and gets five to six hours of sleep on most nights. *"I have to keep my eyes on my goals, but this regimen is exhausting. I need every free minute that I'm not in class or at work to study. But lately I don't have the energy and concentration to study as hard as I used to."*

Target areas: Rasheed needs slow-wave sleep to help clear his mind of useless information and make room for memory consolidation. He also needs Stage 2 to help him with customers at night with his usual energetic and chipper manner.

Nap Rx: One 20-minute "transition" nap after school, before going to his job at the mall; on weekends, a one-hour restoration nap after his shift, before he cracks open his books.

Benefits: Rasheed's weekday Stage 2 naps will help him stay alert and full of friendly good service. His longer weekend nap is for the law student who needs to clear his mind and help him memorize massive amounts of new information daily.

Making it happen: Rasheed now takes his weekday naps (along with other students) in the library at school. He gets to take his weekend nap in the comfort of his own bed and feels that he has almost a four-day weekend, with time to work and study. *"I know I won't be able to keep up this pace forever, but napping has been helping me get through these intense years, staying focused and motivated."*

also the longest, whether we're napping or sleeping. It takes a minimum of 17 minutes before we can transition to our first SWS episode. This dependable phenomenon forms the basis of what is commonly known as "the power nap." The reason this 20-minute wonder leaves you feeling restored and ready to go is that it allows you to reap the benefits of Stage 2 sleep without crossing into SWS and waking up with sleep inertia symptoms (remember, you spend around two to five minutes in Stage 1). Once sleep is underway, each successive appearance of Stage 2 will rarely last longer than eight minutes. In naps longer than 20 minutes, however, you can adjust the proportions of SWS and REM, depending on what time you wake up in the morning and what time you take your nap.

Napping vs. nighttime sleep

I'm often asked if a nap during the day will interfere with nocturnal sleep. The answer is a definite no. Unfortunately, many information sources on sleep hygiene encourage people to avoid napping if they're having trouble sleeping at night. Not only is there not a shred of evidence to support this advice, but much of the data coming out of sleep research demonstrates quite the opposite. In studies across all age ranges, nocturnal sleep duration has been proven to be unaffected by midday napping. As a matter of fact, studies indicate that in a number of cases napping actually improves the ability to sleep at night.

Below are some other questions that may need answering before you begin your nap program.

How long can your nap be and still be called a nap?

To answer this question, it's necessary to examine how the nap functions in terms of our natural sleep cycles, which last around 1.5 hours. If you fall asleep for longer than two full cycles (around three hours), regardless of what time of day or night you do it, you've shot past the nap boundary and into the realm of sleep. After two cycles of sleep (or three hours) you will begin to cut into your nocturnal sleep, since periods of this length disrupt your biologically programmed biphasic pattern, just as a light snack of "a few potato chips" that fails to stop before reaching the bottom of the bag will cut into your appetite for a real meal. Except in cases of extreme sleep deprivation, this kind of "nap gorging" is seldom advisable.

How short can your nap be?

It's interesting to hear people describe what they think is the shortest amount of time beneficial to be asleep. Many insist that once they lie down, an hour or more must elapse before they rejoin the waking world and that getting up any sooner makes the effort pointless. More experienced nappers swear they get all they need in 20 minutes. The truth is, all of us are capable of sleeping in increments much smaller than that. Increments as short as a few seconds, known as microsleep, have been proven to occur in the lab. In order to justify being called a nap, however, the period must extend to five minutes or more. This is the point when scientifically proven and detectable benefits begin to accrue.

How long after waking must you wait before napping isn't simply falling back asleep? How long before your intended bedtime should you conclude your nap?

Obviously, it's common to wake up and fall back asleep once or twice during the night. If you get out of bed at 5:45 A.M. to use the bathroom or get a glass of water and sleep from 6 to 6:45 A.M., the latter segment would not be considered a nap. These periods are what sleep scientists call waking after sleep onset, or WASO, a practice that has become quite common thanks to the invention of the snooze alarm. In order for the nap to be completely disengaged from the sleep process, a period of at least two hours should elapse. On the P.M. end, waking up less than three hours before your anticipated bedtime will interfere with nocturnal sleep.

Can napping ever replace nocturnal sleep?

No. Naps are not meant to be a replacement for a good night's sleep. A nap can help you get the most out of your day (and evening), and people have often been shown to be more productive after a nap than if they'd simply worked straight through the day without sleep. Naps can also offset the most acute effects of sleep deprivation, and under extreme circumstances a strategic napping regimen has been shown to help maintain functioning in the absence of normal nocturnal sleep. Like fasting or endurance running, such a practice may have value when used infrequently and judiciously, but for most people, most of the time, nocturnal sleep is essential.

Is the sleep you get from a nap the same as the kind you get at night?

By most measures, yes. The polysomnograph of a person in the middle of a long nighttime sleep will look identical to that of a person taking a short midday nap. However, some important features do distinguish the nap from nocturnal sleep and justify having separate terms to apply to each. Our circadian clocks are programmed for long sleep during the night and short sleep during the day. So while sophisticated MRIs and polysomnographs cannot tell a nap from a long, deep sleep, a simple thermometer often can. For reasons unclear, nocturnal sleep occurs when our body temperature is at its lowest, while napping

Warning signs

While napping is generally a healthy natural function, in certain cases it can be a symptom of some kind of underlying disorder. Excessive daytime sleepiness is one of the warning signs of clinical depression (which, interestingly, is occasionally treated by keeping the patient awake for 24 hours). People suffering from narcolepsy, a neurological disorder in which the brain cannot regulate normal sleep/wake cycles, can also find themselves needing to nap during the day. Of course, even people sick with the flu or some other illness will find themselves drawn to their beds. However, in all these cases, other symptoms besides merely the desire to nap would be present for such diagnoses to be made.

occurs when our body temperature is at its peak. This means that the quality and quantity of sleep are very much affected by whether you are sleeping in the day or at night. Anyone who has ever tried to sleep for only an hour in the middle of the night can feel the difference in comparison with an afternoon nap. Actually, short sleep in the middle of the night can be less beneficial than no sleep, since nighttime is when you're programmed for long sleep, whereas a nap as short as five minutes during the day can give you a much-needed boost.

Furthermore, as will be demonstrated in the next chapter, napping can be controlled and programmed to provide the precise benefits you need in your life.

CHAPTER 6

Optimized Napping:

the secret formula

W hat time did you wake up? What time will you be taking your nap? The answers to these two simple questions lay the groundwork for figuring out the best nap for you.

The discovery that sleep is adjustable, made by myself and a few colleagues at Harvard University, is the basis for thinking of the nap as a self-improvement tool. All that was missing was a way for the average nonscientific mind to actually compute or determine the content of any given nap. By combining the sleep pressure values and plotting them against the circadian graphs and adding the constant value of Stage 2, I've created a nifty algorithm called the Optimized Napping formula. (It's included in the Appendix, but if you want to play around with it, go to my Web site, saramednick.com.) The calculations behind it are a bit complicated, but this needn't deter you from taking advantage of the results any more than not understanding electricity would prevent you from flicking on a light switch. By using the Nap Chart (more on that soon) and factoring in what you know about sleep pressure and circadian rhythm, you'll get more out of your nap than you ever thought possible.

So now the fun can begin. We'll start by designing two very different naps so you can see how the formula applies to all kinds of lifestyles, no matter how extreme.

The lark and the owl

A ll naps are not created equal. This holds true even if two naps are taken at the exact same time at the exact same length. Let's take a look at two such naps, both one hour long, both taken at noon. Our first napper, Laura, is a "morning person," known in the sleep trade as a lark. She rises and shines at 6 A.M., and though she gets a good jump on her day, so does her sleep pressure. Even without hooking her up to a fancy machine, I can, from my experience in the sleep lab, plot the course of her nap as follows:

> **60% Stage 2 (36 minutes)**
> **17.15% SWS (10.29 minutes)**
> **22.85% REM (13.71 minutes)**

Laura's nap has a good balance between all the sleep stages. She will find she's getting sustained attention and alertness, physical and muscle improvements, recovery and repair of tissue and organs, and extra mental clarity.

On a smaller scale, her nap will contain the following schedule of sleep events:

> **noon to 12:02 P.M.—transition to Stage 2**
> **12:22—transition to slow-wave sleep**
> **12:32—transition back to Stage 2**
> **12:40—transition to REM**
> **12:54—transition back to Stage 2**
> **1:00—wake-up**

Not insignificantly, a nap taken at this time allows Laura to sail through SWS, which ends 30 minutes into the nap, and wake up in Stage 2, thereby diminishing sleep inertia. But this nap cuts it pretty close, since if she let her nap run just five or six minutes longer, she would easily find herself back in SWS and sleep inertia would be a concern.

Now look at Oliver, our night owl. He gets up at 10 A.M. If he naps at noon, the same time as Laura, does he experience the identical nap? Stage 2 is still 60 percent, or 36 minutes, but SWS drops to a mere 8 percent, or 4.8 minutes, and REM rises to 32 percent, or a whopping 19.2 minutes:

> **noon to 12:02 P.M.—transition to Stage 2**
> **12:22—transition to slow-wave sleep**
> **12:27—transition back to Stage 2**
> **12:35—transition to REM**
> **12:56—transition back to Stage 2**
> **1:00—wake-up**

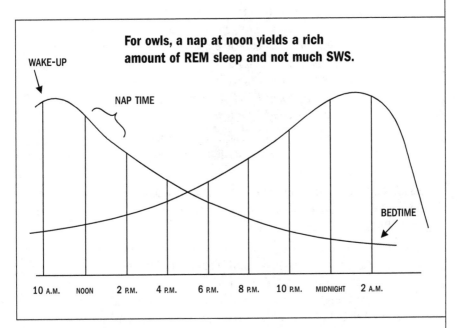

For owls, a nap at noon yields a rich amount of REM sleep and not much SWS.

WAKE-UP

NAP TIME

BEDTIME

10 A.M.   NOON   2 P.M.   4 P.M.   6 P.M.   8 P.M.   10 P.M.   MIDNIGHT   2 A.M.

For creative types, this nap is a powerhouse. Lots of ideas can be generated through naps so heavily weighted with REM. Because perceptual skills also improve markedly with REM, this nap would be great for the visual artist working on fine detail or the proofreader who must catch errors. Conversely, it's lacking in benefits associated with tissue repair and clearing out no-longer-used mental pathways.

Oliver, too, would still easily sleep past SWS but would encounter it again if he were to sleep just five minutes longer.

In order to achieve the same quality nap as the owl's noontime nap, a lark would have to start napping at 8 A.M. Notice, too, that the elapsed time from wake-up in the case of the lark is six hours, while in the case of the owl it's only two hours. Therefore, merely knowing the number of hours after wake-up is not enough to accurately compute the quality of any nap.

A Profile in Napping: **The single mom**

Situation: Natasha, a 38-year-old divorcée raising her 13-year-old daughter, teaches undergraduate courses in art history and is a curator at the art center of a large midwestern university. She sleeps less than seven hours and wakes up at 6 A.M. *"It's hard to meet all the requirements of my job and still be there for my daughter, getting her off to school in the morning, making sure she does her homework and everything else that's involved in raising a child—without help. I'm always feeling rushed, and I'm losing that mental space where I can conceive of more interesting shows to bring to the gallery."*

Target areas: Like any single mom, Natasha needs extra energy and alertness from her nap, but she also must keep the creative parts of her brain from running dry.

Nap Rx: Natasha has two options for her creativity-sparking nap. She can choose the "perfect nap," lasting 90 minutes anytime between 1 and 3 P.M., or a nap at 10 A.M. for at least 30 minutes.

Benefits: The midday nap will give this mom Stage 2 for energy and alertness, SWS to deal with all the information built up in her mind and, most importantly, enough REM sleep to inspire the creative insights she needs to present works of art in fresh and innovative ways. The morning nap will be rich in REM and will provide an added "free association" boost in a limited amount of time.

Making it happen: Twice a week, Natasha keeps office hours on campus between 1 and 3 P.M. Since students don't usually visit except around midterm and finals, she's often able to catch a perfect office-hours nap. On other days, if she heads directly to campus after dropping her daughter off at school, she's able to catch half an hour or more of nap time before class.

A nap to call your own

As illustrated in the foregoing examples, it's possible to examine your nap and learn what stages are contained within it. You can also decide what kind of nap you want—rich in REM, Stage 2 or SWS—and determine the optimal time to take that nap.

The perfect nap

Stack up all possible naps, and there's one clear blue-ribbon winner. This is the nap that occurs under a perfect storm of conditions—the portal in time when your biology is pushing you toward sleep and the environment is piling on as well. In study after study, the majority of subjects, left to their own devices, voluntarily fall asleep when this perfect storm strikes.

Prime napping time, as most people intuitively sense, falls between 1 and 3 P.M. This is when the sun is high and the temperature peaks. According to researcher Roger Broughton, it's also when the rise in our drive to go back to sleep is least compensated by the other levels of our circadian cycles. He called this period "the nap zone." If you nap when the clock strikes the zone and ride it for 90 minutes, you score a nap that couldn't be more optimal in its balance of stages:

5% Stage 1
60% Stage 2
17.5% SWS
17.5% REM

Notice that SWS and REM are present in equal proportions. This distribution occurs only once every 12 hours—at 1 P.M. and again at 1 A.M. It isn't significant during nocturnal sleep (at 1 A.M. we'd likely be in the middle of it), because over the course of all the cycles the stages adjust and balance out anyway. But the thing that makes this the "perfect nap" is that it's like a Mini Me of sleep. In a single cycle, it mimics the overall stage percentages of nocturnal sleep in a fraction of the time.

Studies have shown that this nap can even produce the same benefits as a seven-hour night of sleep. But before you abandon your bed at night and live off your "perfect nap," keep in mind that such a nap can only be this productive in well-rested people who haven't built up a mountain of sleep pressure.

The customized nap

Now, what happens if you need extra REM but your schedule only allows for a late afternoon SWS-rich nap? For instance, if you're an artist with a day job and want to practice your art after you get off work at 5 P.M., how should you calculate your nap? In this case, you can extend your napping time an extra half hour to double up on your REM. Or what if you're a postal worker who's engaged in repetitive, detail-oriented tasks and requires extra SWS but can only take a nap in the early part of the day, when it would be rich in REM? Here again, an extended nap might be in order, or conversely, since SWS always precedes REM, two short naps of 25 to 30 minutes each would provide a short SWS boost before REM sets in. And finally, if you want to avoid waking up in SWS and thus minimize sleep inertia, you can use the Optimized Napping formula to plot your nap across time and learn how to avoid this condition.

As a rule of thumb, you can count on naps earlier in the day to be richer in REM, while late afternoon naps tend to be higher in SWS. If you take particular interest in your dreams, waking up during or right after a heavy REM episode will allow you the greatest recall of your dream imagery. If you feel like one of "the walking tired," a heavy SWS dose will take care of that. Or review the benefits outlined in Chapter 3 and again on page 97 in Chapter 8, decide what you really want out of your nap and then find the corresponding time in your own personal schedule when such a nap can be created. You have that power. Use it.

The Nap Chart

The table below is based off the Nap Wheel, available in an interactive format at saramednick.com. These calculations are based on normal sleep/wake schedules and accurately reflect the concentration of stages only in people who aren't excessively sleep-deprived. Once you're sure that you're in the healthy sleep zone, you can use the chart to design and refine your nap so that it delivers the benefits most important to you.

Remember that the "perfect nap" is 90 minutes long. When creating your custom naps, they should not extend past 3 hours in duration.

Wake-up Time	Perfect Nap Start Time	Prioritize Creativity (REM-Heavy) Nap Start Time	Prioritize Memory (SWS-Heavy) Nap Start Time
4:00 am	12:45 pm	6:00 am — 12:45 pm	2:15 pm — 5:00 pm
5:00 am	1:00 pm	7:00 am — 1:00 pm	2:30 pm — 6:00 pm
6:00 am	1:30 pm	8:00 am — 1:30 pm	3:00 pm — 7:00 pm
7:00 am	2:00 pm	9:00 am — 2:00 pm	3:30 pm — 8:00 pm
8:00 am	2:30 pm	10:00 am — 2:30 pm	4:00 pm — 9:00 pm
9:00 am	3:00 pm	11:00 am — 3:00 pm	4:30 pm — 10:00 pm
10:00 am	3:30 pm	12:00 pm — 3:30 pm	5:00 pm — 11:00 pm

A few final notes are in order here. The formula's calculations are based on the behavior of well-rested people with a normal sleep schedule in a normal environment. While Optimized Napping can generally predict the patterns of human sleep, allowances should be made for human variability as well as other factors. Extremes of temperature, for instance, will artificially shorten REM episodes. If you allow yourself to become chronically sleep-deprived, sleep pressure will become overly heavy and SWS will crowd out the other stages. This is not to say that you shouldn't nap if you're

A Profile in Napping: **Two jobs, one nap**

Situation: Maria works nine to five as a customer service rep, answering phone calls and filing complaint reports. She wakes up at 7:30 every morning. Three nights a week, she takes on a seven-to-midnight waitress shift, and on those nights she gets no more than six hours of sleep. *"I feel like my whole life is work. I would like to spend more 'quality time' with my husband, but he works as many hours as I do. Frankly, we're both too tired to appreciate the time we do have together. On weekends, we usually just crash out."*

Target areas: Maria needs stamina to keep going through her "mindless" day job, her physically demanding restaurant shift and beyond. Getting less than six hours of sleep at night leaves her sleep-deprived and damages her body. Her need for SWS is acute.

Nap Rx: A 45-minute nap every day after work.

Benefits: Stage 2 sleep will give Maria the extra boost she needs, while the extra SWS will help to heal more than just her sore waitress calves. Because of her added sleep pressure, it will take her longer than normal to sleep past SWS and avoid sleep inertia, especially when she must go off to her second job. By relieving that pressure, she will restore her body to a healthy state and her weekend sleep won't be all about catch-up, so she and her husband will have more time to focus on each other.

Making it happen: Since her office provides a protected parking lot, Maria can feel comfortable taking a nap in her car after work. On free nights, there's always the couch at home.

sleep-deprived. The point here is that your body will use these naps to repay your sleep debt. As you catch up, you can start experimenting with more sophisticated and cutting-edge tools of the nap technology. Eventually, as you work in tandem with your Sleep Profile (see Chapter 7) and become more internally aware of your own passage through the stages, you can wean yourself from the generalized formula. Then you can create an even more precise style attuned to your particular and idiosyncratic rhythms—a nap that is truly all your own.

Part Three:
The Program

Your sleep profile:

getting to know yourself

Context is everything in the study of sleep patterns. Before I begin an experiment, I need to know what my subjects have been doing, thinking and feeling for two weeks beforehand. Without this information, it would be impossible to tap the nap's full potential.

That's why, in this chapter, I'm going to ask you to become your own sleep scientist. By taking a few moments each day over the next two weeks to inventory your habits, your coping strategies, your weaknesses and strengths, you will be laying the foundation for greater wellness and productivity. The questions you are about to answer have been adapted from actual sleep study assessments, designed to track the relationship between your sleep habits and the areas of your life most affected by them. The truth is, sleep does not exist in a sealed container cut off from the rest of our physical, mental and emotional being. It interacts with almost every other aspect of who we are and what we do, yet few of us are aware of what goes on moment to moment in our lives unless we are specifically instructed to pay attention. Sure, you could start napping today, but by first creating a framework around which your nap can be properly understood, you can harness the force of that nap to create the maximum amount of positive change in your life.

So get ready to be reintroduced to a very special person: yourself.

How tired are you?

Before getting into your daily assessment, it's important to determine your level of daytime sleepiness. The Epworth Sleepiness Scale below asks you to rate how likely you are to doze off in a variety of circumstances. Even if you haven't done a particular activity, try to estimate the likelihood of dozing while doing it (or something similar). Use the following scale to choose the responses that best apply to you:

0 = Would never doze
1 = Slight chance of dozing
2 = Moderate chance of dozing
3 = High chance of dozing

SCORE	SITUATION
	Sitting and reading
	Watching TV
	Sitting inactive in a public place, e.g., in a meeting or a theater
	Riding in a car as a passenger for an hour without a break
	Lying down to rest in the afternoon
	Sitting and talking to someone
	Sitting quietly after lunch (when you've had no alcohol)
	Sitting in a car while stopped in traffic
	TOTAL SCORE

Interpreting your score:

A score of less than 8 indicates normal sleep function. For active and alert people who score less than 8, a nap will be an enrichment tool, a means of adding up to a second "whole day" (in terms of mental clarity and overall stamina) in the middle of your day or just ramping up your alertness and cognitive and/or motor skills.

A score of 8 to 10 indicates mild sleepiness. For people scoring in this range, a nap will not only create a second day but also will clear away any daytime sleepiness that can prevent optimal performance.

A score of 11 to 15 indicates moderate sleepiness. People scoring in this range should be concerned that their sleepiness may interfere with daily activities, concentration, relationships, and so on. (People receiving treatment for sleep apnea usually score about 11.7.) A nap will be an essential tool in creating a healthy lifestyle.

A score of 16 to 20 indicates severe sleepiness. People scoring in this range should speak to their physician about testing for a sleep disorder, while also being sure to take regular naps. (People with untreated sleep apnea score about 16.0; people with narcolepsy, about 17.5.)

A score of 21 to 24 indicates excessive sleepiness. People scoring in this range may suffer from a severe sleep disorder.

Remember, nobody is beyond improvement. Let your score be your personal starting point on the road to positive change.

Checking your calendar

Why, you ask, must you make a note of everything you eat or drink, the length of time you spend working, what your mood is like or what you're thinking about, just so you can start napping? You'll never know how far you've come unless you know where you've been. So, for a two-week period, use the calendar to track your habits, answering the questions either in the morning or evening as indicated. In doing so, you'll not only be attuning your-self to the aspects of your life most affected by sleep, but you'll create a baseline from which to assess your improvements. Later on, you can test yourself again and see how far you've come. To follow your progress, you can download the chart from my Web site, saramednick.com.

YOU AND YOUR SLEEP

To be answered in the morning:

1. What time did you first try to go to sleep last night?

2. How long did it take you to fall asleep last night?

3. Did you need a sleep aid? Type and dosage?
   (Include nonprescription and herbal formulas.)

4. How many times did you wake up during the night?

5. What time did you wake up this morning?

6. How many total hours of sleep did you get last night?

7. Did you feel refreshed upon awakening?

YOU AND YOUR LIFESTYLE

To be answered before going to bed:

8. How many cups of caffeinated beverages did you consume?
   When?

9. How many alcoholic drinks did you consume? When?
   How much? (1 drink = 12 oz. beer, 1.5 oz. liquor, 5 oz. wine)

10. Do you take any other medications? (These include
    nonprescription medications, recreational drugs and herbal
    supplements.)

11. Did you smoke? How many cigarettes per day?

12. Did you exercise today? What time? For how long?

13. Did you experience bouts of sleepiness during the day?
    What time(s)?

14. Did sleepiness interfere with your day's activities?

15. Did you nap today? When? For how long?

16. Rate on a scale of 1 to 5 how refreshed you felt when you
    woke up from your nap (1 = the lowest, 5 = the highest).

HOW DID YOU FEEL TODAY?

Rate the following areas of your life on a scale of 1 to 5
(1 = the lowest, 5 = the highest):

How was your mood today?

Your overall alertness?

Your overall stamina?

Your overall mental abilities?

Your physical health?

The quality of your interactions with friends and family?

Now comes the fun part that every scientist lives for: interpreting your data. By having your most important indicators tabled out in front of you, you can easily determine which aspects could use some strengthening and which only need to be maintained. With these findings as a baseline, you will then be able to set realistic goals for yourself.

The questions to ask yourself when looking at your profile are divided into three sections: 1) you and your sleep, 2) you and your lifestyle, and 3) how do you feel?

You and your sleep

In this section, you evaluate the amount, consistency and quality of your overall sleep.

How much sleep are you getting each night?

The amount of nocturnal sleep you get is the most fundamental element in any sleep profile, since it has the greatest impact on all of your wellness indicators. Studies have shown that sleeping eight hours a night will give you the full spectrum of benefits. Seven hours is considered adequate. Drop below that and you begin to "starve" your body and will likely notice repercussions during the day. And anything less than six hours will set off alarm bells as your biological systems go into disaster mode, increasing insulin levels, blocking the consolidation of memories and making you feel downright lousy.

While there is no replacement for sufficient nocturnal sleep, a nap can help minimize or reverse these effects.

What time are you going to sleep at night? Does that time change as the week progresses?

Become more aware of whether you're maintaining a regular bedtime schedule and know that the optimal bedtime is somewhere between 10 P.M. and midnight. It's common to find yourself going to bed at a reasonable hour on Monday and then watch bedtime slowly creep into the later hours as the week progresses. As you've already learned, the first part of the night is dedicated to the most restorative kind of sleep. By falling asleep later, you rob yourself of a balanced sleep diet.

This can be partially corrected by napping. And with the benefits of sustained concentration, alertness and stamina, you might even discover that you accomplish more in your day so the nights don't need to get so late.

Are you spending a lot of time trying to get to sleep?

If you use sleep aids, do you see a particular pattern?

How many times do you need to get up at night?

Difficulty with getting to sleep or maintaining sleep can be due to many different factors, and we employ a variety of strategies— from counting sheep to swallowing pills—to deal with it. Ideally, you would like to be completely free from artificial sleep aids and still sleep peacefully for a solid 7.5 to 8 hours, getting up at most twice in the night. Periods of restless sleep can occur in everyone due to temporary stressors, but a chronic problem needs to be brought to the attention of your physician. Since there are many excellent treatments for sleeplessness, nobody has to live without nature's balm. But for now, be aware of whether certain days are more "sleep difficult" than others. Napping can decrease your feelings of fatigue and stress so that you might find it easier to sleep at night. See to what extent this is true for you.

Is there a big difference between your total sleep time on weekdays and the weekend?

Playing weekend catch-up is a strong indicator that you're not getting enough sleep during the week (this is particularly true among teenagers who habitually sleep past noon on Saturday and Sunday). Between Monday and Thursday, does your nocturnal sleep drop from a healthy eight hours to a dangerous six? This is common under Type A Fallacy conditions, when you think you can accomplish more by sacrificing sleep. The problem is, although you might sleep from Friday night straight through into Saturday (or crash out all day on Sunday), the damage has already been done. People usually report feeling worse after sleeping excessively (over 10 hours in a 24-hour period)—the so-called sleep hangover. Try going to bed between 10 P.M. and midnight on weeknights; on weekends, shift these times by no more than an hour. This keeps your biological rhythms steady and won't throw you for a groggy loop every time you have to reset your clock on Monday morning. See how that affects how refreshed you feel when you wake up. And as you integrate napping, notice how that affects your weekend-to-weekday sleep balance. This will also tell you whether you use napping to make up for lost sleep or to enhance your already well-rested self.

Do you have difficulty adjusting to your weekday schedule? Is waking up on Monday difficult?

In the same way that you limit variation in your bedtimes, your wake-up times should remain as consistent as possible to achieve a healthy sleep lifestyle. Shift workers, especially those who work irregular and inconsistent hours, show greater health problems than their coworkers who have more traditional working hours. Try and adjust your wake-up times so they're within an hour or two of one another across all days of the week. This means that if you wake up for work between 6 and 8 A.M., you should get up no later than 9 A.M. on Saturday and Sunday.

One tip is to try easing a nap into your schedule on a Monday, and see if that doesn't help cushion the blow of the weekend-to-weekday shift. You may even find yourself looking forward to Monday, since you know you won't be dragging yourself through the whole day.

You and your lifestyle

This section addresses the effects of sleep on other aspects of your daily life.

Do you notice a change in your caffeine intake?
What about cigarettes, alcohol or other drugs?
How often do you snack between meals?

Fatigue has been shown to be closely linked with drug and alcohol abuse, so it's important to be aware of whether your need for stimulants and depressants increases as your sleep decreases. Sleepy people are also more likely to reach for fattening snacks throughout the day in order to boost flagging energy. For example, some people tend to get less sleep on Thursday night than on Monday night, and, not surprisingly, they will drink more caffeine at work as the week progresses and be more likely to hit the local happy hour afterwards. Others find that the number of cigarettes they smoke rises as the week draws to a close.

Be aware if any of these statements are true for you. Ideally, stimulants should not be needed at all, but if you smoke, it stands to reason that you'd like to smoke less and quit sooner. If you must have coffee, you can limit it to one or two shots in the morning. Caffeine stays active in your system for up to seven hours, so keep this in mind as you try to implement a daytime nap. Also, remember that caffeine comes in all shapes and sizes. Your need to reach for that Diet Coke at lunch or when that 3 P.M. slump comes around could signal that caffeine is the crutch you're using to drag yourself through the day. Watch what happens to your caffeine intake when you exchange your 15 minutes at the coffee cart with a little shut-eye at your desk. How many cigarettes do you smoke then? Have you cut down on snacking? How do these changes affect all your other habits? As you become more awake and alert, note the wiser choices you make about what you put in your body and feel good about them.

What time of day do you get the most exercise?
How do your exercise habits affect your sleep?
Everyone knows that exercising at least 20 minutes (ideally, more) several days a week improves cardiovascular fitness. But regular exercise is also recommended to help you sleep well. The timing of the workout, however, is important. Low body temperature is good for nocturnal sleep, so if you exercise late in the day and have trouble falling asleep, try moving your regimen earlier than four hours before bedtime to give your body a chance to cool down. For

napping, on the other hand, high body temperature is optimal, so a post-workout nap can be just what the doctor ordered and an easy solution for nappers in training.

Is there a specific time during the day when you always get tired? Is there an increase in the amount of daytime sleepiness as the week progresses?

As you know, a dip in the afternoon occurs in all of us. Is this when you start feeling tired? What happens to your productivity and mood during this time? Perhaps you will discover that you might as well be asleep for all the mistakes and lack of focus you experience during this bewitching hour. How do you usually cope with this dip? Does the dip become more apparent as you move from Monday to Friday? Your ability to handle the afternoon slump decreases the more sleep-deprived you are. Once you've implemented your nap, you may find that it actually becomes your magic hour. Notice whether you perform better and what your energy level is like in the afternoon and evening.

How do you feel?

This is the most subjective part of the profile, asking you to fill out a "report card" rating your performance in various areas. Sleep-deprived people will generally score between 1 and 3 in these evaluations of mood stamina and mental energy. They are often too tired for quality time with friends and loved ones and lose the desire for intimate relations with their partner. You will likely notice that your moods are closely correlated with the amount of sleep you get. No amount of artificial stimulants will erase this effect. You'll find that they only make things worse.

Napping during the day will elevate your mood and give you a lot more energy that you can share with your loved ones. You might even discover that napping with your partner can improve the relationship!

Different naps for different folks

I t bears repeating: There's no such thing as a bad nap. Any time you spend in midday sleep will reduce the effects of fatigue and bestow benefits. But our nap needs differ across populations and will change over the course of our lives. A mother's requirement is not the same as that of her three-year-old toddler. The sleep profile of a middle-aged football coach had little in common with that of a teenage beauty contestant.

Let's look across the spectrum to see how every stage of life demands its own particular nap response.

Changes in sleep across the life span

From childhood through early and late adulthood, we see dramatic decreases in SWS and REM.

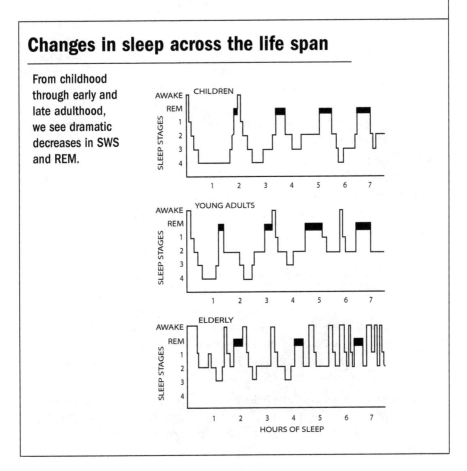

Infants: sleeping machines

As a first-time mother, Julie is surprised to find that her son, Eli, is sleeping 16 to 18 hours a day in his first month of life. But at this early stage, when Eli's brain is undergoing the greatest developmental changes it will ever experience, life is all about sleeping (and feeding). Two basic types of sleep emerge: quiet (non-REM) sleep and active (early REM) sleep. Not surprising, active sleep predominates, since the power to acquire new skills and behaviors runs off the REM battery. Over 50 percent of neonate sleep is active

A Profile in Napping: **The parent trap**

Situation: Liam and Neha are twentysomething working parents with a toddler and a newborn. They average less than six hours per night of sleep and often get less than four. Liam works full-time as a software engineer, and Neha's maternity leave will last only three months. *"After Rebecca was born 18 months ago, the amount of sleep we got plummeted. We were finally getting back to normal when Sunshine was born. This time around, we're feeling that it might get a bit overwhelming."*

Target areas: For three months, all bets are off for long periods of core sleep. Neha will obviously be the major carrier of this burden, but Liam will be involved as well. All aspects of their functioning will be impaired; getting as much sleep as possible whenever opportunity allows is critical.

Nap Rx: Ideally, an afternoon nap, around 3 P.M., of at least 45 minutes. But the parents must also grab sleep wherever and whenever possible.

Benefits: The 3 P.M. nap normally delivers around 20 minutes of Stage 2 sleep, approximately 15 minutes of SWS and maybe a dash of REM. Liam and Neha are sleep-deprived, so SWS will undoubtedly muscle in on their REM time. That's okay, though, because their most critical needs are for Stage 2 sleep to maintain alertness and SWS to relieve sleep deprivation symptoms. Extra REM is a luxury that will have to wait until the kids are off to school.

Making it happen: Both Liam and Neha learn to sleep when the baby does. Neha in particular lets go of the notion that she should try to get things done during this time, so now when Sunshine drifts off, mom does, too.

(premature babies can achieve levels as high as 80 percent), but that number will drop to 30 percent by the end of the first year.

An infant's sleep begins to level off at around 14 to15 hours by the fourth month and remains there for the next four months. Some parents may notice that their babies have a reversed pattern, sleeping longer during the day than they do at night. This is common and will eventually shift to a more normal cycle. Other infants may take longer to segregate their sleep into predictable intervals, and parents are left to find a way to work around this erratic schedule as best they can.

Early sleep cycles spin more rapidly than those of adult cycles, coming back to REM every 50 to 60 minutes. By age two, however, REM will occupy 20 percent of total sleep, as it does throughout childhood, adolescence and adulthood. Napping emerges a little before the end of the first year, when sleep coalesces into a nocturnal sleep period, a shorter nap (a half-hour) in the morning around 10 A.M. and a longer one (1 to 3 hours) in the afternoon around 1 or 2 P.M.

Toddlers: nap, wake, repeat

Two-year-old Sarah needs to sleep about 12 hours out of 24, but she's also beginning to become aware of herself and has learned the word "no." Stalling or refusing to go to sleep at the prescribed bedtime becomes more of a problem. This type of behavior occurs in about 10 percent of the childhood population. But social structure will have a greater influence on her sleeping and eating activities once she begins preschool. The long days of social interaction will cause her to look to bedtime as a welcome opportunity for rest. Studies have shown, however, that not getting enough sleep can make children more difficult at bedtime. Once again, napping is the solution. Children who are not irritable and exhausted when nighttime comes around will actually take to bed more willingly. And remember this: At the age of two, only 8 percent of children nap

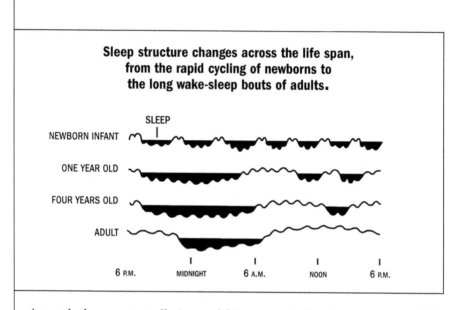

Sleep structure changes across the life span, from the rapid cycling of newborns to the long wake-sleep bouts of adults.

irregularly or not at all. Around 25 percent will take two naps, while the rest will take one long nap.

There is a slow decline in sleep needs—about 30 minutes per year—starting at the age of one. By age five, a child needs between 11 and 12 hours of sleep out of 24, almost all of which can be achieved at night. But if you notice signs of fatigue, reintroduce an afternoon nap as a transition between school and home life, or ask your child's teachers whether they can make a place where he can take a nap during school. But do not let your child sleep too long (over three hours) or too late in the day (two to three hours before bedtime), or you'll have difficulty getting him back to sleep at a normal hour.

Children: losing it vs. using it

Children between the ages of 5 and 13 need 10 to 11 hours of sleep, but during this stage of their lives napping starts to go out of style. (Sleep time goes down about 25 minutes per year between ages 5 and 10.) Only 17 percent of kids between the ages of 5 and 8 take naps; by puberty, only 9 percent do. Many kids use the weekends to catch up on sleep, demonstrating that it's not so much sleep needs that are changing; rather, too-early school start times are getting in the way of sufficient sleep. Catch-up sleep is okay in temporary situations, but it should not be encouraged on a regular basis.

There are many forces working against good sleep health among children, with caffeinated and sugared drinks being prime culprits. Cutting down on these drinks and hopefully eliminating them from your child's diet can produce a surprising increase in her ability to take a little nap after school or before homework or evening activities. As she gets older and participates in more extracurricular events, explain to her that she can improve her stamina, as well as her ability to learn, with even 15 minutes of scheduled nap time before band practice or soccer. Ways to encourage this include giving her an extra 15 minutes in the car on the way to the next activity or getting her to a location early so she can take a nap in a warm, safe place before the activity begins.

Adolescents: ch-ch-changes in rhythm

Teenagers actually require more sleep than adults—about nine hours—but often get much less. With earlier school start times, sports, after-school jobs and whatever it is they're doing when they say they're over at a friend's house, most teenagers usually manage 6.5 to 7 hours of sleep on weeknights and then "crash" on the weekends, sleeping 10 to 12 hours Friday and Saturday nights to make up for the accumulated debt. To complicate matters, adolescents experience a timing delay in their biological clocks that causes a similar lag in the timing of sleep onset. Thus teenagers naturally tend to go to bed later and sleep through the morning—the very thing parents don't want them to do!

All of the above factors have resulted in a sleep debt crisis that has only one solution: napping. This will be tough for some parents, but if your teenage child collapses on the couch upon returning home from school, embrace the habit and let him sleep for an hour or so. He's making up for sleep deprivation while consolidating the full load of information from classes, sports and social interactions. Part of the task of helping kids understand the changes caused by the onset of puberty is to let them know that their biological clocks are undergoing a transformation that can cause them to feel full of energy one moment and then tired and deflated an hour or so later. Explain the basics of sleep hygiene, including avoiding caffeine and keeping a regular sleep/wake schedule. And establish the two-hour rule. If they're in bed by 11 P.M. during the week, 1 A.M. should be the latest they can go to sleep on the weekend. The same goes for waking up.

Teenagers who can't seem to fall asleep before midnight or 1 A.M. should be encouraged to nap during the day so they can be sure to get as close to nine hours of sleep as possible. One family found that getting their teenage daughters to nap was one of the only pieces of advice they didn't argue with!

College-age napping: an introductory course

Jeff is a 26-year-old neuroscience grad student. "As an under-graduate," he says, "I would think nothing of staying up all night to study, but I don't like to put myself through that anymore. Once I started napping, I learned I could fall asleep when I wanted to and wake up ready to read stacks of articles, finish my written assignments and even function optimally during exams." For his daily nap ritual, Jeff has a very specific system: "I sit at my desk, listening to music with headphones on and fold my arms in my lap. I keep my head down a little so it doesn't nod. I always wake up after 15 minutes."

Napping for students, especially during midterms and finals, is absolutely essential. Student nappers usually have an eye for the best spots on campus: the library because it's quiet, or the student lounge with its big, comfy couch. Unfortunately, it's becoming a trend on campuses across America to remove couches from these places in order to discourage students from napping! Considering the amount of research in favor of napping and the health risks of going without sleep, it's time for campus activists to insist on the students' right to nap.

The middle years: early waking, late napping

Hany was recently promoted to the chair of the Department of Computer Science at an Ivy League college. He has no trouble falling asleep at 11 P.M. every night, but no matter how tired he is, he can't sleep past 2 or 3 A.M. Whether he rolls around in bed or putters around the house, he doesn't fall back asleep until 4 A.M. Then he sleeps till 6:30 A.M., when he has coffee (but no breakfast) while catching up on e-mails and the news. He's at work by 9 A.M. and by mid-afternoon he's dead-tired. Still, to get everything done, he stays on campus until 8 or 9 P.M.

At age 37, Hany is a victim of a sleep phenomenon that many men approaching middle age are familiar with: early morning waking. His nap must address the buildup of fatigue due to sleep deprivation as well as facilitate the massive amounts of multitasking and problem-solving he does all day. The perfect nap for him is a mid- to late afternoon nap around 3:30 P.M., lasting around an hour. This nap will provide 20 minutes of Stage 2, 15 minutes of slow-wave sleep and a little less than 10 minutes of REM. His wake-up time coincides with the REM episode, so he's guaranteed to wake up feeling refreshed and ready to tackle the tasks ahead. Stage 2 provides a boost for the mid-afternoon doldrums, reversing any patterns of deterioration in his motor skills from typing all day, reading and doing detailed work. Fifteen minutes of SWS will clear away bits of useless information built up across the day, and that sprinkle of REM that ends the nap allows him to avoid sleep inertia.

As Hany ages, both SWS and REM will diminish. He may also report that his nocturnal sleep is less satisfying, due to an increase

Are men's naps from Mars, women's from Venus?

Nocturnal sleep hours average about the same for both sexes (6.7 hours during the workweek and 7.3 hours on the weekends), but recent evidence suggests that men take more naps than women do. Men spend more time awake in bed and enjoy less slow-wave sleep and REM, but this doesn't mean that women do not have problems sleeping. They just begin later in life. A recent study showed that young women fell asleep faster and overall had better-quality sleep than their male peers did. The young men also reported more daytime tiredness than the female subjects.

As women mature, they report more problems with insomnia than men do and are more likely to use sleeping pills. One large gender gap in sleep results from the hormone roller coaster that females undergo throughout their lives. For instance, a National Sleep Foundation poll found that 51 percent of pregnant and recently pregnant women reported at least one weekday nap; 60 percent reported at least one weekend nap. Pregnancy can bring on disturbed sleep, most severely in the third trimester, with more awakenings and shallower SWS. Postpartum, sleep efficiency falls to an all-time low, so new mothers rarely get into the deep, restorative SWS and also suffer a decrease in REM. To make matters worse, they experience a drop in their threshold for auditory stimuli (the level of sound needed to bring you out of sleep) as well. According to the National Sleep Foundation, 47 percent of women aged 40 to 49 experience difficulty sleeping, and the figure climbs to 50 percent when they reach age 50. Among other things, sleep disturbances, including insomnia and sleep apnea, are frequently reported complaints among menopausal women; some experts estimate that a woman may wake up hundreds of times a night due to hot flashes. Fortunately, women are learning about the benefits of exercise, regular bedtimes and wake-up times, dietary changes and improved sleep environments.

Now, who really needs a nap more: a man or a woman? They both do.

in his trouble falling asleep and increased sleep fragmentation or awakenings. Pressures such as these, and the relief supplied by a little bit of midday sleep, lead many people to first "discover" the nap when they hit their 40s and 50s.

The golden years:
napping for the actively retired

The sleep of seniors is fragmented and "light." What is lost with aging is the consolidation of the sleep state and the "deepest" delta (Stage 4) sleep. In addition, the internal clock tends to advance in the elderly, so it's not unusual for a 70-year-old to go to bed at 7 or 8 P.M. and wake up at 4 or 5 A.M., unable to return to sleep. People over the age of 65 also find it difficult to stay awake between 1 and 4 P.M., and this is when they're at the greatest risk of falling asleep at the wheel.

If you're a senior with nocturnal sleep problems, your nap will be a wonderful way of fighting the dangers of excessive daytime

---

A Profile in Napping: **The golden-year triathlete**

Situation: James is a 52-year-old semiretired electronics engineer and active triathlete whose wake-up time is 5 A.M. His schedule varies according to the sport he's training for that day. *"On swim days, I go swimming for 45 minutes and spend 15 minutes in the sauna. On bike days, I go for a 2-to-3-hour ride and don't come back until three or four in the afternoon. On run days, I'll also run for two to three hours. Since I'm not as young and limber as I used to be, I need every advantage I can get."*

Target Areas: James needs two things from his nap: an energy boost and a restorative tonic for his hardworking muscles.

Nap Rx: A 20-minute nap at 1 P.M. on swim days; a longer, 45-to-60-minute nap at 3 P.M. after bike rides and runs.

Benefits: The 20-minute naps, all Stage 2, are super for stamina, motor performance and alertness. The 45-minute naps help to restore muscle tissue with a rich dose of SWS after a strenuous bike ride.

Making it happen: James takes his napping as a serious part of his triathlete training, especially before any kind of competitive event. *"Once my nap is over, I have the second part of my day with my wife at dinner or the movies or just relaxing at home."*

sleepiness. If nighttime sleep isn't a problem for you, I recommend the Ultimate Nap (see page 49). Remember to double-check what time of day your Ultimate Nap will occur, since you may be waking up earlier than you did in your youth and therefore your Ultimate Nap opportunity will present itself earlier as well.

CHAPTER 8

Nap time:

it's easier than you think

All humans are biologically programmed to nap, but the demands of modern life have driven this natural impulse into hiding. Some people even insist that they're physically incapable of napping! So how is it that even the hardest cases suddenly nap like babies when they're brought into the lab?

The answer lies in the physical, psychological and social conditions that go along with the experimental milieu. In the lab, subjects are told they're *allowed* to nap. They're provided with a comfortable space with controlled noise and climate, separate and distant from the stressors that prevent sleep. On top of that, they're given detailed instructions that include not only a method of falling asleep but also a careful list of activities and substances to avoid. I'm going to show you how to duplicate that experience wherever you may find yourself—minus the electrodes, of course.

Certainly, clinical insomnia, sleep apnea, asthma, rheumatoid arthritis or any other chronically painful disorder can disrupt sleep and require medical intervention. However, none of these conditions acts solely upon the nap. If you have little or no trouble falling asleep at night, by following the simple guidelines in this chapter you *can* nap.

It's about time

"Who's got time to nap?" is a common complaint among non-nappers. The short answer is: just about everyone. If you spend 20 minutes or more at Starbucks getting an afternoon mocha latte, couldn't you just stay where you are and take a nap instead? So, before you conclude that napping doesn't fit into your busy life, take out your day planner and examine your schedule. By carefully reviewing the activities of your day and the time it takes to do them, you can assess which time expenditures are unnecessary and where a nap can be substituted. How long is your lunch? A paralegal with an hour lunch break reports that she can eat in half an hour and keep the second half for her nap. Or do what I do and pencil in 20 to 40 minutes as soon as you get home for a transition nap between work and leisure.

Once you've carved out those precious minutes, you need to make this nap time a regular feature of your day. Just as we've developed a detailed trail of cues for our minds and bodies to recognize that it's time for nighttime sleep, we need to fashion a similar set of cues that will indicate that it's nap time. Consistent scheduling allows the body to associate that hour with the nap and all other concerns to more easily fade away.

Clearing the way

While it's true that people have been known to fall asleep almost anywhere, some places and some conditions make it easier than others. It's important to identify and remove any "nap blockers," especially those associated with work or other responsibilities. Doctors, put away your stethoscopes. Handymen, take off those tool belts. And students, hide those textbooks. Minimizing learned psychological stimuli and crafting a dedicated nap space—even if it's a foot away from your desk—will create a buffer between the pressures of life and your improvised nap sanctuary.

Safety first

Many of us could not imagine a peaceful nighttime slumber without a dead-bolt lock and high-tech alarm systems to protect us from the outside world. So let's apply these security considerations to the nap. For instance, if your place of employment has secure parking, consider napping in your car. (Remember during the summer months to keep your windows cracked.) Or if you choose to nap in the park on your lunch break, you should feel secure that your belongings will not be interfered with or that you won't get rudely awakened by a soccer ball to the head.

Be mindful not just of your own safety but of everyone else's as well. If you decide that the best place to take a nap is under your desk, be sure you're out of the way of passersby who might accidentally trip over your feet. On the other hand, you can make all that human traffic work for you. For her noon nap, Karen, a 45-year-old creative director of a boutique advertising agency, unrolls a foam mat and positions it so that if the door opens, it hits her feet and wakes her up. "It's my natural alarm clock," she says. Since her coworkers are used to her napping schedule, the "alarm" seldom rings before she gets her full 45 minutes.

Hold all calls

On location, the actor Jeff Bridges often retires to his trailer and hangs a NAPPING sign on the outside so he won't be disturbed, but less glamorous workplaces still have a way to go before that level of nap consciousness takes hold. The trick is to focus on what is actually under your control. The announcement we hear in movie theaters, lecture halls and libraries requesting that we silence all cell phones, beepers and other electronic communication devices should certainly be observed when it comes to napping. If your computer is close by, put it into sleep mode, too. There's plenty of time to find out if "You've Got Mail" once you wake up.

Let there *not* be light

Amy is a 36-year-old single mother with a special-needs child who wakes her up at least a couple of times a night. "I was never able to nap," she recalls. "Even if I missed a night's sleep, I could never nap the next day." But now Amy has had to *learn* how to nap. "I started using one of those eye pillows with seeds in it," she says. "People think you're supposed to put it right on your eyes, but most of it actually goes on your forehead and it kind of droops down to your eyes. I began using some yoga techniques, too, but getting that little pillow is what really put me over the edge. After all these years, I've learned that my primary nap blocker is light."

Nappers of yore managed to avoid sunlight easily enough, but the invention of the lightbulb presented daytime sleep with a pernicious challenge—at least in those cases where the switch is not under our control. The culprit, biologically speaking, is melatonin. Produced in the pineal gland, this hormone acts upon the hypothalamus, which causes the brain to switch into sleep mode. (As an

Lights out

Sleep shades comes in a variety of fabrics, ranging from basic airline polyester to soft pillowed silk. Pay attention to the breathability of the fabric. A cotton weave will cause less stickiness and heat buildup. Look for a brand with nose clips and ear loops, as opposed to one that has to be tied to the back of your head; these keep the shade in place when you shift positions. A good pair will run you anywhere between $10 and $20.

Pay a little more, and your nap can be enhanced by, say, an Aromessentials Sleep Mask with Lavender-Chamomile Scented Sachet from Dream Essentials (dreamessentials.com). Or, if money's no object, consider a hydrating sleep shade that keeps your eyes (and contact lenses!) from drying out as you nap. Bucky Products (bucky.com) even offers a velour sleep shade with a pocket for storing your earplugs (included).

artificial supplement, 3 milligrams of melatonin has generally proven effective at ameliorating such sleep aberrations as jet lag and even insomnia.) Light inhibits the production of melatonin, and that's why it's easier to fall asleep in the dark. To keep those levels up, close the blinds, shut the lights and, if all else fails, invest in a sleep shade that covers your eyes.

Quiet, please . . .

Close your eyes and tune in to the sounds of your environment. What do you hear? Most likely, plenty. The world has become a very noisy place. The EPA cites a nighttime average level of 35 decibels (quieter than the hum of most refrigerators) as conducive to uninterrupted sleep. Laws, not to mention rules of courtesy, prevent major eruptions of sound in the middle of the night. Airplane traffic is redirected to comply with residential area noise limits. Loud parties prompt calls to the police, and without a pressing emergency no construction crew would dare begin operations before the sun comes up. But afternoons—as many would-be nappers learn to their chagrin—are a sonic free-for-all.

Sleep interference is not simply a matter of decibel levels. Sound is produced in waves. Matching a wave with its opposite creates an effect called noise cancellation, or "white noise." Because white noise contains all frequencies, it can be used to mask other sounds; our ears are trained to pick out specific frequencies, not to respond to overall sound level. Many people would be surprised to learn that the volume in an airplane cabin hovers around 110 decibels, nearly as loud as a rock concert. But we are generally unaware of this racket because it's hidden in plain "earsight" as white noise. Devices known as noise cancelers artificially create these matching waves and are the high-tech method of choice to create a quiet sleep environment.

Of course, thousands of people have achieved the same result using earplugs, which range in construction from foam to plastic, rubber, down or silicone and are priced accordingly from 25¢ to $300 a pair. The most expensive variety can be used on land or in the water, are molded to fit your own ears and feature acoustic filters that provide protection against high-level impulse noises from 140 to 190 decibels. Hard to believe, but the maker of Insta-Mold earplugs promises super-soft hydrophobic silicone plugs that can change color or glow in the dark! Test several brands for yourself and compare their effectiveness, comfort, durability and price.

Keep in mind that the NRR (noise reduction rating) listed on most packages can be a good guideline, but the figures are based on lab tests. As with your car's MPG, your actual mileage (i.e., sound blocking) will vary.

Temperature: degrees of napping

You might be surprised to learn that scientific research pinpoints a slightly nippy 65 to 68 degrees Fahrenheit as the optimal temperature for sleep. But this is only a prescription for long nocturnal sleep, which is triggered by low core body temperature. While it's almost always true that napping is biologically the same as any other kind of sleep, the one qualitative difference is that while nocturnal sleep occurs at the icy pole of our core body temperature cycle, napping most frequently occurs at the balmy equator. So keep the thermostat at a comfortable setting, or add a coat or blanket. Light blankets work better than heavy ones, since some people report that getting too warm and cozy has led them to oversleep their allotted nap time. Keeping yourself slightly cooler makes it likely that you'll wake up from REM, so this is a good option for those who want to nap for around 40 minutes.

To make napping easier when you're away from home, consider purchasing a fleece blanket and yoga mat that can roll up together with a handy strap; these can be found at most travel or camping stores.

Proper posture

When it came to napping, Winston Churchill insisted that there should be "no halfway measures." "Take off your clothes," he said, "and get into bed."

While the convenience of a nearby bed might have been available to the British prime minister, such luxuries are seldom within the reach of the rest of us. However, our bodies associate certain stereotypical postures with sleep, and approximating these as closely as possible will assist in getting you into that mode. If there is no place to lie down, at least raise your feet. For one jet-setter, the ability to sleep in a fully reclined pose was so important that she spent hundreds of extra dollars for an upgrade to business class. If your budget precludes such extravagances, at least lean back and make sure your head and limbs are well supported so your body can maintain its position even after the muscle paralysis and relaxation that accompany sleep onset. Otherwise, you can fall victim to the "nap nod" often observed on public transportation when people are jerked awake by their head falling forward.

Pillow talk

Nap pillows come in all shapes and sizes. Depending on your nap position, you might want to choose a roll pillow, possibly with a built-in pocket for a cool or warm compress. Or try the designer NAP pillow available from Brookstone, made with microbeads for a softer, more malleable headrest.

Travel pillows are good to have when you're on a train, plane or bus. While the inflatable ones are the most convenient (they can store flat and then be inflated in a few breaths), they are often poorly designed to fit the contours of your neck and can cause all kinds of kinks and cramps. A better choice is a pillow made with heat-sensitive "memory foam," which will fit your neck shape no matter what position (sitting up or lying down) you happen to find yourself in. The cost will be somewhere between $15 and $50.

The cutting edge

Science has done more than simply come up with more precise nap techniques; it has helped to launch a consumer revolution in sleep products. So, unlike the creative thinkers of centuries past, who relied on tricks to wake themselves up from their naps, you can avail yourself of an array of exciting products that use the latest technology to create a more restful nap.

1. "Shake Awake." An innovation in wake-up technology, this vibrating alarm clock sends powerful pulsating vibrations to noiselessly wake up the sleeper. It's pocket-size, so it's the perfect thing for public napping or for nappers who are hard of hearing or who want to avoid the stress of a loud electronic wail ringing in their ears.

2. "SleepSmart." By incorporating the technology of polysomnography, which reads the electrical signals of your brain to determine your sleep stage, this alarm clock can be programmed to wake you up when you're in a lighter sleep stage and eliminate sleep inertia for good.

3. "Sleep-Eze." If ordinary earplugs don't meet your standards, for a mere $200 or so you can buy an in-ear white-noise machine that will electronically cancel all outside noise.

Drugs and diet

In the sleep lab, caffeine intake is carefully controlled. Few people would drink a cup of coffee at 11 P.M. unless they were planning a late night at the office, at school or out on the town. You have to apply that same rule to your nap. Translation? No caffeine up to four hours before you expect to sleep. And beware of stealth stimulants. Caffeine lurks in tea, chocolate and many of your favorite soft drinks and so-called "energy elixirs." Recently, a young female research subject slept for only 20 minutes out of the hour-and-a-half nap time allotted in the study. When questioned, she revealed that she had mistakenly ordered a Diet Coke because she "had one for lunch every day."

4. Light-stimulation alarm clocks. These clocks incorporate the science of melatonin and the body's response to light, waking you up gently with a "dawn simulator" that slowly increases levels of light. For a few dollars more, get the optional sunset simulator (to aid in falling asleep), too.

5. Sound pillows. Now, along with the great advances in pillow construction, you can have your own personal soundscape (from music to crashing waves) emanating from tiny speakers embedded in a comfortable pillow and attached to a CD player, without the awkwardness of wires and headphones.

6. "Dream Helmet." This is the device that ties it all together—a sleep mask and sound-blocking pillow and pockets to keep your valuables secured all rolled into one headgear. Perfect for the traveling napper.

As always, caveat napper! A new product with all kinds of fancy bells and whistles won't necessarily do anything to improve your nap experience. More often than not, the manufacturer's claims will not have been seconded by hard scientific data. A case in point is a "neuro-linguistic" audio device whose manufacturer claims only that its benefits are "theoretically possible." This is not to say that music or other sounds cannot induce napping, but before you shell out $150 for an unproven technology, see if you can't get the same or better results from your favorite relaxing music on a $10 CD.

Nicotine is another central nervous system stimulant that can interfere with the natural sleep process. Although its effect varies depending on how many cigarettes are smoked, nicotine can stay active in the bloodstream from one to two hours. This makes it difficult to nap during that time.

In addition, many prescription and over-the-counter medications such as ephedra (a common cold medicine ingredient), diet pills, antidepressants, nicotine patches and other products that ameliorate nicotine withdrawal all interfere with the natural sleep rhythm. Of course, many people require these drugs and have been prescribed them by their doctor; in such cases, scheduling a nap between doses will allow the action of the earlier dose to dissipate and the next dose can be taken upon waking.

Ironically, even depressants accompanied by warning labels about driving and operating heavy machinery can become nap blockers. Fragmented sleep (interruption or shortening of the natural sleep cycle), which typically occurs when sleeping off depressants, interferes with the ability to nap by throwing the body's rhythms out of whack. Let's take the most common depressant: alcohol. You can easily fall asleep after a three-martini lunch, but then the alcohol transforms into a kind of stimulant and wakes you up before your body is completely refreshed. What sleep you *do* get lacks the benefits that accompany drug-free slumber; in other words, all it does is process the drug out of your system. So the likelihood is that you will feel less clear-headed upon waking than you did before you started drinking! This is not a lecture about the dangers of drink. Just be aware that everything you put in your body affects your sleep/wake—and nap—cycle.

Certain foods can also function as nap blockers. Sugar should be avoided prior to napping; the "sugar high" will keep you buzzing instead of sleeping. Refined sugar, which delivers the quickest and purest jolt of energy is, of course, the worst offender. (Under ordinary circumstances, even carbs—bread, pasta, potatoes—quickly break down into simple sugars and can have a similar, though less intense effect.) Foods high in saturated fat content require a lot of digestive work, and the subsequent indigestion or heartburn can get in the way of your nap. So watch the fast food before nap time. And finally, too much liquid or any kind of diuretic will interfere with continuous sleep . . . for obvious reasons.

Does this mean nappers must go hungry? Certainly not! Hunger is a surefire wake-up trigger. So what's left to put on your plate? Protein. It's broken down slowly in the body and offers long-term sustained energy. Foods such as turkey, cheese and nuts are high in the amino acid tryptophan, a precursor to melatonin, and actually promote sleep. Calcium helps the brain synthesize melatonin from tryptophan, so adding milk, cottage cheese and yogurt to your menu makes these foods work even better. Other nap-friendly foods include tofu, soy milk, soybean nuts, seafood, lean meats, poultry, whole grains, beans, rice, hummus, lentils, eggs and sesame seeds. Truly a napper's feast!

Free your mind and your nap will follow

Even with a diet free of stimulants and an environment where conditions are optimal, some people still might find that they're unable to nap—largely because of the noise in their own heads. If you have internalized negative beliefs or attitudes, it doesn't matter how careful and meticulous your nap preparations have been—you might as well be trying to nap in the middle of a busy intersection. It's time to confront this beast head on by identifying the most common varieties of a syndrome we call cognitive nap aversion, or CNA. This syndrome refers to the thoughts that prevent your body from following the normal pathway to sleep. The solution is a three-pronged attack: Identify, Address, Replace.

1. Identify. Before you can make any headway as a napper, it's important to recognize any negative attitudes or beliefs that stand in the way of your nap and how you came to have them.

2. Address. Once a particular mind-set is exposed, you can "treat" it with clinical and research-based information. Only then will you be able to understand that your misperceptions are neither factual nor helpful.

3. Replace. Having cast off your misperceptions, don't just leave your mind in "neutral." Fill that old mental space with a more positive associative set.

Below are some of the most common psychological nap inhibitors. If any of them sound like something you've heard yourself say . . . well, you know what to do.

"If I nap, I'm being lazy."

Some of the most hardworking figures in history—national leaders, scientists, CEOs, movie stars—have used napping as a tool to get more out of each day. As demonstrated by the latest brain imaging technology, your mind is still at work even if your body is at rest.

Replace with: **"Napping makes me more productive."**

"I'm too busy to nap."

Just look around your office at 3 P.M. More than likely, instead of a hive of industrious activity, you'll see a bunch of bleary-eyed workers checking and rechecking their e-mail. As the great napper Winston Churchill said, "Don't think you will be doing less work because you sleep during the day. You will be able to accomplish more. You get two days in one . . . well, at least one and a half." The latest scientific research has proven him correct.

Replace with: **"I'm so busy, I need to nap."**

"I haven't done enough to deserve a nap."

Do you deserve to eat? To breathe? No natural function—including napping!—should be regarded as a privilege. Stop cheating yourself.

Replace with: **"I'm exercising my inalienable right to nap."**

"I can't get anything out of a 20-minute nap, so why bother?"

You can reap benefits in as little as five minutes. Naps under 20 minutes can increase alertness, improve physical dexterity, boost stamina and lower stress. Post-lunch naps of 15 minutes have been shown in university studies to increase alertness and performance.

Replace with: **"In less than 20 minutes, I will restore my alertness for the rest of the day."**

Okay, you're cleared to nap!

As a beginner, don't be worried if napping doesn't come easily on your first try. Remember your first time at the gym? That wasn't a banner day, either. It's been a long time since your early napping days, and you're out of practice. Don't put any additional pressure on yourself. This is not an Olympic sport, and no panel of judges will be grading your performance.

Review what you've already learned about Optimized Napping in Chapter 6 and how it applies to your individual needs. Below is a reminder of the benefits of each sleep component to help you in using your Nap Chart.

	THE BENEFITS
STAGE 2	• Reduced sleepiness
	• Heightened alertness
	• Increased concentration
	• Enhanced motor performance
	• Elevated mood
SLOW-WAVE SLEEP (SWS)	• Clearing of useless information
	• Improved conscious memory recall
	• Restorative tissue repair
RAPID EYE MOVEMENT (REM)	• Increased creativity
	• Improved emotional memory
	• Keener perceptual and sensory processing
	• Better memory of complex associative information

Over the next two weeks, allow your nap regimen to stabilize. Count off the days to build anticipation of the improvements you'll discover during your next assessment two weeks from now.

Still awake? Read on . . .

Like anything else that requires a relaxed mental and physical state, napping will become more elusive the more effort you put into it. The trick is to be able to get out of your own way and let your body do what it does naturally.

To help that process along, I suggest an approach based on the idea of systematic desensitization, which involves not only gently getting the physical body used to the series of behaviors and processes involved in napping but also uncoupling unpleasant or anxious feelings conditioned from previous experiences or ideas. This is helpful for nap newbies as well as ex-nappers who somehow lost the habit and are having trouble reconnecting to their old lifestyle.

Begin by simply lying down or sitting back. Close your eyes. (If you don't feel comfortable closing your eyes, that's fine; leave it for later.) Deepen and lengthen your breathing patterns—shoot for five-second inhales and five-second exhales. If napping feels really strange to you, you can start by simply imagining yourself napping during the day in a pleasant, nonthreatening environment. Also, if at any time you feel vulnerable, afraid or uncomfortable, you can back up until you feel assured that all is well and then ease back into the sequence.

Start by doing this exercise for five minutes daily, then add a few minutes more each day. Don't worry about falling asleep. Just lie there or sit back until you feel a little more relaxed than when you started. Keep at it, pay attention to your nap blockers and, most important, make yourself feel good about what you're doing. You are now creating a web of positive associations around this activity and diminishing the negative ones. Within a few days, you will more than likely fall asleep and wake up without being aware of it. Microsleep—

short, early-stage sleep—occurs commonly under these conditions. In the lab, people woken up during this period will insist they haven't been sleeping, even though their EEGs clearly show otherwise.

So look behind you. Without realizing it, you probably just crossed an important threshold on the way to becoming a napper.

16 steps to sleep

As a final nap aid, try the clinically proven relaxation exercises outlined in the following pages. You can use them every day in your nap regimen or simply on those occasions when you find it more difficult than usual to fall asleep.

This technique involves tensing and relaxing muscle groups one at a time in a specific order, generally beginning with the lower extremities and ending with the face, abdomen and chest. The entire sequence should take you 20 to 30 minutes the first time; with practice, you may decrease this to 15 to 20 minutes. You might want to record the exercises on an audiocassette to expedite your early practice sessions or purchase a professionally made tape of progressive muscle relaxation exercises. In any case, after a week or two of practice, many people find that they can do it from memory.

You can practice this technique seated or lying down. If possible, wear comfortable clothing, and try it out in a quiet place free of all distractions. Keep track of your breathing throughout each exercise, inhaling as you contract each muscle group and exhaling as you release the tension. Ideally, you should breathe from your abdomen. (Begin with a few practice breaths, feeling your abdomen expand and your chest rise as you inhale.)

Hold each contraction for 7 to 10 seconds, then relax. While releasing the tension, try to focus on the changes you feel when the muscle group is relaxed. Imagery may be helpful in conjunction with the release of tension, such as imagining that stressful feelings are flowing out of your body. Give yourself 10 to 20 seconds to relax between each exercise.

The 16 steps have been divided into four muscle groups. You may find that one group needs more attention than another. By identifying these areas, you will open the door to becoming a more relaxed person overall.

Ready? Let's begin:

I: LOWER EXTREMITIES

1. Tighten your buttocks by pulling them together. Hold . . . then relax. Imagine the muscles in your hips going loose and limp.

2. Tighten the muscles in your thighs all the way down to your knees. (You might have to tighten your hips along with your thighs, since the thigh muscles attach at the pelvis.) Hold . . . then relax. Feel your thigh muscles smoothing out and relaxing completely.

3. Tighten your calf muscles by pulling your toes toward you (flex carefully to avoid cramps). Hold . . . then relax.

4. Tighten your feet by curling your toes downward. Hold . . . then relax.

II: TORSO

5. Tighten your shoulders by raising them up as if to touch your ears. Hold . . . then relax.

6. Tighten the muscles around your shoulders by pushing your shoulder blades back as if to touch them together. Hold . . . then relax. Since this area is often especially tense, you might repeat the sequence.

7. Tighten the muscles of your chest by taking a deep breath. Hold . . . then exhale slowly. Imagine any excess tension in your chest flowing away with the exhalation.

8. Tighten your abdominal muscles by sucking in your stomach. Hold . . . then relax. Imagine a wave of relaxation spreading through your abdomen.

9. Tighten your lower back by arching it. (You should omit this exercise if you have lower back pain.) Hold . . . then relax.

III: HEAD AND NECK

10. Tense the muscles in your forehead by raising your eyebrows as far as you can. Hold . . . then relax. Imagine your forehead muscles becoming smooth and limp.

11. Tense the muscles around your eyes by clenching your eyelids tightly shut. Hold . . . then relax. Imagine sensations of deep relaxation spreading all around your temples.

12. Tighten your jaws by opening your mouth so widely that you stretch the muscles around the hinges of your jaw. Hold . . . then relax. Let your lips part and allow your jaw to hang loose.

13. Tighten the muscles in the back of your neck by gently pulling your head way back. Focus only on tensing the neck muscles. Hold . . . then relax. Since this area is often especially tight, it's good to repeat the tense-relax sequence.

IV: UPPER EXTREMITIES

14. Clench your fists. Hold . . . then relax.

15. Tighten your biceps by drawing your forearms up toward your shoulders and "making a muscle" with both upper arms. Hold . . . then relax.

16. Tighten your triceps—the muscles on the undersides of your upper arms—by extending your arms out straight and locking your elbows. Hold . . . then relax.

Stay motivated!

Again, don't expect miracles. The most profound and durable changes in life take place slowly. Be patient with yourself. And stick with it. Periodically repeat your two-week assessment to give your health regimen an occasional tune-up and gain an even greater perspective on your progress. From your first nap to your 10th nap to your 110th nap, this little resource will never stop delivering better health, a cheerier mood, more brain power and extra stamina. Instead of constantly needing more to get the same level of benefit, as people tend to do with chemical helpers, you will actually start spending *less* time napping because you've learned how to fall asleep at will and your nap has become more efficient. As any veteran napper can attest, it only gets better over time.

You can make your adventure in sleep wellness more interesting and fun by inviting your spouse, a family member or a colleague to participate with you. Touch base with them regularly for mutual encouragement and support. Solicit advice from your doctor, dietician, therapist or exercise coach. They can often be a source of support and inspiration. Don't worry if you miss a day or two. Just get back on the schedule. Failure comes not to those who suffer lapses or mistakes, but only to those who quit trying. And remember, there are no "right" or "wrong" answers. This is not a competition. Nobody can disqualify you or vote you off the island. And everybody who enters wins. The prize: a newer, better, happier you. Enjoy!

CHAPTER 9

Extreme napping:

exploring the outer limits

"*G*etting thrown around a bit right now. It's quite violent . . . haven't slept for more than 20 minutes in one go, and probably 15 minutes on the first night and maybe a couple of hours total in the last 24 hours. . . .*"*

—FROM A SHIP'S LOG KEPT BY ELLEN MACARTHUR

Ellen MacArthur sails on the edge—of sleep science. In 2001, she captured the title of fastest woman to sail solo around the globe. Then, in February 2005, she circled the planet in 71 days, 14 hours, 18 minutes and 33 seconds, breaking the previous world record by more than a day and becoming the fastest human to perform this feat, period. Accomplishing this giant leap for womankind required sustained attention to course direction, weather conditions and more. With mountainous seas, giant icebergs and gale-force winds to struggle against, even four hours of core sleep could result in disaster (as it was, her ship nearly collided with a whale!). That's why MacArthur's victory was one not only of seamanship but of human endurance. Out there, the old rules just don't—or can't—apply.

When it comes to exploring the limits of the nap's power, MacArthur has quite a lot of company. Billionaire adventurer Steve Fossett has piloted himself around the world in every kind of craft imaginable, sleeping very little in the process. In February 2006, Fossett completed the longest nonstop flight in aviation history, flying 26,389 miles in around 76 hours, subsisting only on five-minute power naps and his specialized milk shakes.

Any self-respecting sleep scientist must hasten to add, "Don't try this at home." There is no real substitute for adequate core sleep. But sometimes, in extreme situations, napping is all we can do. Think of soldiers in battle, firefighters in a raging blaze, rescue workers after a catastrophe, a hospital in a crisis. For them, nocturnal sleep is simply not an option. Even under less heroic circumstances—say, a project with a harsh deadline—people may find it impossible to get their healthy nocturnal sleep.

In the world of biology, staying awake for weeks is not unheard of. Migratory birds, following their own deadlines, pull this off on a biannual basis, flying thousands of miles without letup. The internal mechanisms that allow them to do this are also available to a lesser degree in human beings. Now, we too will journey beyond the healthy everyday sleep regimen to answer the question, "How far can I push my nap, and what is the most effective way to do it?" Please use this information responsibly.

Überman to the rescue?

Extreme sleep schedules have been practiced since the time of Leonardo da Vinci, an experimenter himself with eccentric sleep styles. Few people have done more to advance the knowledge of the practical applications of this technique than Harvard sleep researcher Claudio Stampi. In the early 1980s, Stampi conducted many rigorous tests of human endurance by regulating sleep/wake schedules. Vigilance and decision-making tasks were continually monitored to determine the minimum amount of sleep needed to maintain optimal performance over the longest period of time.

Stampi eventually pioneered a system called polyphasic ultra-short sleep that involved a series of 20-to-120-minute naps and no core sleep over periods that could last for weeks. Moving his program from the laboratory to the sea, he refined it in conjunction with more than 100 sailors in oceanic competitions. When coupled with the adrenaline of competition, carefully managed lack of sleep proved to induce a mental state that enabled sailors to accomplish feats that they would be incapable of duplicating under normal circumstances.

The polyphasic sleep program has many variations, but the general practice requires dividing the day into three parts. By catching one 90-minute cycle during each 8-hour "mini-day," subjects were able to maintain maximum performance levels despite the fact that their total sleep time was only 4.5 hours per 24-hour period. If pressed for even more time, it's better to shorten one or more of the naps but always maintain the 8-hour day. In fact, situations like competitive open-sea racing call for nap sessions of 20 minutes or less at times! This strategy produced the most winning teams in Stampi's study, even though other strategies involved more rest—sometimes as much as 3 or 4 hours more per each 24-hour period.

Like some kind of pharmaceutical drug that finds its way to the street, polyphasic ultrashort sleep has turned up in college dorms and on the fringes of the Web as Überman napping. Offering themselves up essentially as guinea pigs in the study of sleep deprivation, students and others have adopted a lifestyle of napping for indefinite periods and posting their experiences on the Internet. Before you, too, throw caution to the wind, remember that even under the best of circumstances, such a program is not sustainable over a long period and does not provide the full package of benefits enjoyed by those with proper sleep schedules. Going ultrashort is like running a marathon or climbing Mount Everest. You need careful training and a generous period of recovery. Without professional guidance and supervision, you'll likely fail to reap the benefits of the extra hours that you seek and you may do yourself some damage besides. One of Stampi's most critical findings was that the motivation of individual subjects is a key determinant in how well they're able to adapt to a sleep-starved diet. Thus, ultrashort sleep works best when it's practiced by highly motivated individuals who are engaged in focused, goal-directed behavior, as opposed to the Über-man nappers who just passively observe their own reactions to this unusual physical state.

As a scientist, I appreciate the opportunity to read through the case studies posted online. But as someone more concerned with the health and cognitive benefits of napping, I cannot recommend the lifestyle. Suffice it to say, quite a few of these sleep outlaws' narratives end with "I quit after I got sick."

Still, it's clear that the more sleep-deprived you are, the worse it is to sleep monophasically. Instead, frequent bursts of work followed by short periods of rest is the most efficient way to maximize human ability in times of sleep scarcity. If you find yourself in such a situation, the golden rule might appear counterintuitive: sleep less. Getting yourself to the point where less is more, however, is often the hardest part. Polyphasic ultrashort sleep requires three to five days—sometimes more—of preparation to get your system in sync with the new schedule.

Living without core sleep is a little like being launched into outer space. The laws of nature don't quite behave in the ways we would expect. For instance, the stages of sleep (1, 2, 3, 4, 2, REM, 2, 3, 4, 2, REM . . .) suddenly appear randomly like songs on an iPod set on shuffle. REM might appear before Stages 3 and 4, and indeed in the absence of those stages, or it may be obliterated by slow-wave sleep. And Stage 2, the trusty constant that normally precedes and follows SWS and REM, can disappear and leapfrog the napper directly into REM. After a few days, order is established within the chaos and the proportional relationship between the

---

A Profile in Napping: **The impossible deadline**

Situation: A week from now, Andrew, a 26-year-old Web designer, will receive
material from which to create a site that would normally take between two
and three weeks to complete but for which he's been given only a week and
a half. A night owl, Andrew typically wakes up between 9 and 10 A.M., but
he'll soon face little more than 4 hours' sleep per each 24-hour period.
*"I usually just slog through without sleeping and make up for it later, but my
work certainly does suffer. I need to find a smarter way to get through those
10 days."*

Target areas: In extreme situations, fighting off the worst effects of fatigue and
keeping alertness up to safe levels is the critical task.

Nap Rx: Immediately insert a 1.5-hour nap around 3 P.M. Wake up one to two
hours progressively earlier each day (larks who wake up at, say, 6:30 A.M.
should simply go to bed an hour or two later) and slowly add more naps.
During the "10 days of hell," when Andrew is actually building the site, he
should maintain a strict pattern of 6.5 hours awake and 1.5 hours asleep.

Benefits: Andrew's rhythmic sleep schedule creates balance between his sleep
stages, and he's better able to focus the extra adrenaline that results from
his efficient sleep management as well as his general level of motivation.

Making it happen: Before Andrew tackles the assignment itself, he prepares his
body for ultrashort sleep. He likes to sleep late, so waking up earlier each
day requires a strong will and a loud alarm clock; the effort, however, pays
off. *"I found the transition week difficult, but when it came time to perform,
I felt almost as if I was launched out of my bed and into my work."*

---

stages, when added up over a 24-hour period, will be the same as in
normal nocturnal sleep.

So, if you foresee a no-sleep zone ahead, start modifying your
sleep a few days before it hits. Or, failing that, expect a bit of a
"learning curve" as your brain and body adapt and adjust to the new
sleepless reality.

Although it's almost always better to get a long dose of core
sleep, when that's not possible, you must resist the urge to "nap
gorge." Thus, while the choice between taking a 90-minute nap or

a 180-minute nap might sound like a no-brainer, especially when you're dead-tired, the latest research suggests you opt for the former. That's because 90 minutes will take you through a full cycle of sleep and bring you out in REM or Stage 2 sleep, allowing you to avoid sleep inertia, which at this point in your sleep deprivation would be quite severe. Studies comparing subjects deprived of core sleep who received one cycle of sleep with those who got two found no difference in performance. In this unusual case, the time is actually better spent in work or study than in sleep. Again, this holds true only in short-term situations—no more than two weeks. Over the long haul, more sleep wins out every time.

If you can manage it, schedule your 90-minute nighttime nap between 1 and 3 A.M. During the afternoon, shoot for sometime between 1 and 3 P.M. These, as you recall, are the "perfect nap" zones, where nap cycles will be ideally balanced between REM and SWS.

Finally, after putting yourself through such exertions, it's just as important to give your body what it needs on the way down. Polyphasic sleepers build up a massive sleep debt, and the SWS pressure can be immense. Because SWS needs must be satisfied before REM can reassert itself, expect up to two near-dreamless nights of deep sleep recovery, followed by two nights of epic dreaming as you experience an equally long rebound of REM. It isn't necessary to crash for 12 hours during the recovery period. By giving yourself 8 hours of core sleep and a generous 90-minute nap in the middle of the day, you will smoothly return your system to balance rather than swinging from extremes of not enough sleep to too much sleep. On the fourth day, when your sleep finally returns to its normal pattern of stages, get back to your usual healthy habits and your regular daily nap. Remember: Your body is engineered to pull out all the stops when it comes to short-term superhuman feats. But as with taking a loan from a good friend, it's okay in times of dire need; abuse that generosity and you'll likely find your friend less giving the third or fourth time around.

Napping for "normal" emergencies

Even if you'll never pilot a craft around the world or even have to work for weeks without letup, at one time or another you'll probably be called upon to stay up for a night, a weekend or a few days to accomplish some task. What kind of milder nap solutions are available for those temporary crunch times?

Your choices in this regard can be broken down into three categories, each with its own scientific designation.

1. The preventive nap. This is the nap we take in anticipation of an extended period of sleeplessness. Preventive naps work to extend a period of alertness and stamina and serve to stave off the symptoms of fatigue. The drawback of such naps is that they have an early "expiration date." The beneficial effects cannot be expected to last past 8 to 10 hours.

2. The operational maintenance nap. This is the nap taken during the work period in anticipation of fatigue but before any symptoms of performance decline become manifest. Consider this your "workhorse nap" in your hour of need. By stealing away for a 20-minute Stage 2 nap whenever possible, you can maintain your alertness without having to deal with sleep inertia. An extended nap would keep you going longer, so either make use of one of the sleep-inertia minimizing techniques (e.g., bright lights, a splash of water) or, better yet, nap your way past SWS, being sure to wake up well before its second coming (between 50 and 90 minutes is a pretty safe bet), so you can benefit from *all* the sleep stages.

3. The operational recovery nap. This is the nap you take after fatigue has already caused your performance to deteriorate. Research demonstrates that this technique should be used only as the nap of last resort. Why is this so? Because "an ounce of fatigue prevention is worth a pound of recovery." Once sleep deprivation sets in, you make your sleep work harder. Of course, this doesn't mean you simply skip your nap. You only become a greater danger to yourself and others the longer you are sleep-deprived. Remember: It's never too late to prevent a fatigue-related mistake.

Graveyard-shift workers face a slew of dangers. By forcing the body to stay awake when it naturally wants to sleep and making do with sleep when the body normally feels it should be awake, there is an increased risk for cardiovascular and gastrointestinal disor-

---

A Profile in Napping: **The convention crunch**

Situation: Chris, a 32-year-old junior partner in a technology firm, needs to be at his best all weekend for an important convention. He'll get only three and a half hours of sleep per night. *"The pressure is really intense. We leave work in Los Angeles on Thursday and fly to Las Vegas, check into our hotel and then immediately set up. We man the booth in the convention hall during the day, and afterwards there are motivational meetings to attend and 'hospitality suites' to host. My energy and enthusiasm has to always be at its highest. Over 25 percent of the company's new business is generated at these events."*

Target areas: Concentration, altertness and stamina. Also must stave off effects of acute short-term sleep deprivation.

Nap Rx: A preventive nap of at least 40 minutes before reaching Las Vegas. Once the convention is in full swing, at least one 20-minute "power nap" per day. Afterwards, return to a stable pattern of seven to eight hours of core sleep and a short afternoon nap.

Benefits: The preconvention SWS nap will stave off sleep pressure as long as possible, while the Stage 2 Chris gets from his operational maintenance naps will keep his alertness going without any sleep inertia so he can immediately go back out onto the convention floor and be at his sharpest.

Making it happen: Chris knew that the flight time would almost certainly be spent strategizing with the other partners, so he took a 20-minute nap before the airport van came to pick him up. In Las Vegas, the hotel convention center offered numerous "nap nests" for Chris to sneak off to for quick 20-minute power naps between presentations and meetings.

ders, plus greater vulnerability for obstructive sleep apnea. The propensity of these workers to make errors on the job is greater than that of their daytime counterparts. They're more likely to fall asleep at work and their drive home, statistically speaking, is the most dangerous commute of all workers. Science has yet to determine whether these conditions are the result of staying up all night or simply the poorer quality and shorter duration of sleep that graveyard-shift workers get. Still, the issues that need to be addressed are sleep deprivation and the restoration of balance to their normal hormonal cycles, which have been badly disrupted.

Operational napping is most critical for workers on the graveyard shift. Studies have shown that, on average, shift workers sleep for 1.5 hours less a day than permanent day workers. By taking a quick 20-minute Stage 2 nap, they're able to recharge their essential alertness skills and stave off the most hazardous aspects of sleep deprivation. Since they will still suffer symptoms associated with graveyard work, they must try to schedule an hour nap sometime during the day. Note that because of the disruption of natural circadian cycles in this kind of work, the rules of the nap formula will not apply.

Adjusting to a nonfluctuating shift is easier, since the circadian phase will eventually adapt to a permanent change in the routine. In other words, the REM cycle will move to the new "night," which might in fact be in the middle of a sunny day. But many workers alternate among three shifts, so their circadian rhythms have no chance of keeping up. Not only are these people sleeping at different times every day and usually significantly less than non-mixed-shift workers, but the major environmental cues that usually help keep the circadian cycles tuned—sunlight, noise, social interactions and alarm clocks—are also inconsistent. It is simply impossible for the body to synchronize with them, so any sleep is fragmented and often not restful. Naps taken as a preventive strategy will help supplement the much-needed sleep in this population.

Even if we don't work "extreme" hours, our jobs can throw our natural rhythms out of whack. Lily, for instance, is a chef at a fast-paced New York City restaurant. Although she is not naturally an owl, her chosen profession has caused her to take on later hours as her prime "on" time. "I have to get to work at 4 P.M. to start designing the dinners and organizing the prep," she says, "so I'm out of my apartment at 3:15. This means I need to be awake by 2:45 P.M. It would be great to take a nap sometime during work, but the floor of a busy kitchen is no place for a rest period. I need to find another solution."

Lily is a prime candidate for the preventive nap, since its effects don't have to last past her shift. It just has to take place as

A Profile in Napping: **The graveyard shift**

Situation: Married with three sons aged 6 to 14, Wayne works 10 P.M. to 6 A.M. He falls asleep at 8 A.M. and is lucky to go six hours before waking. *"I thought this schedule would be ideal, since I'd be able to spend time with my wife and kids. But daytime sleep is hard—there isn't much peace and quiet. I get irritated easily, and it's hard for me to enjoy my time with my family."*

Target areas: Wayne needs extra alertness and must also defuse the buildup of sleep pressure. The symptoms associated with graveyard work, such as poor health, sleepiness, irritability and increased accidents, need to be addressed.

Nap Rx: A 20-minute operational nap during the night shift; a one-hour nap sometime around late afternoon. *Note:* Because of the disruption of natural circadian cycles in graveyard-shift workers, the rules of the nap formula will not apply.

Benefits: The Stage 2 power nap will recharge Wayne's alertness battery. The midday nap will be heavily weighted with the SWS he needs to counter the effects of sleep deprivation.

Making it happen: Instead of taking advantage of the vending machine snacks, Wayne now lies down for a nap during his midnight break. Twice a week, when his kids have after-school activities, he helps himself to another nap at 4:30 P.M., an hour before everyone gets home. Since he doesn't have to be at work until 10 P.M., the occasional sleep inertia from SWS-heavy sleep isn't much of an issue.

close to the start of work as possible. Lily now naps for 1.5 hours beginning at 1:15 P.M. after a healthy light lunch. After a shower at 2:45 (this washes away any sleep inertia), she's ready for a long night of chopping, sautéing and reducing.

For "owls" and others forced to work early shifts, the prescription is the same except that they should take a recovery nap in the afternoon when they get home from work. This way, they still have the evening (naturally their most productive time) to be alert and awake.

Napping across time zones

Nothing plays more havoc with your circadian rhythm than jet travel. While a lot of "experts" insist that napping exacerbates jet lag, this is not necessarily true. The essential "fix" needed to recover from this common nuisance has to do with getting your system regulated to a new night-and-day cycle. This means sticking to your customary schedule, including seven to eight hours of nocturnal sleep and a healthy daily nap. Napping should be avoided outside of your normal regimen because it will throw off your body's attempt at self-regulation. But a well-placed nap can also help you through the out-of-sync feeling that comes from a disrupted circadian clock, especially in circumstances where you need to be alert and productive at your destination.

Needless to say, don't abandon all the tenets of jet lag avoidance. Stay hydrated throughout the flight and avoid alcoholic beverages. For the few days prior to your departure, be sure to keep to a regular sleep/wake schedule, but go to sleep 15 to 30 minutes earlier each night if you're traveling east or 15 to 30 minutes later if you're traveling west. Once at your destination, you'll want to help your body adjust to the new time zone by continuing your regular sleep pattern—including your nap taken at your regular time. You might find that 3 milligrams of melatonin at night will help "shift" your biological clock to coincide with your new surroundings.

The hypnogogic nap:
skimming along the surface of sleep

Why did so many artists, scientists and inventors clutch a fistful of spoons, ball bearings or coins when they nodded off? The answer is that they knew their muscles would relax and the objects would crash to the floor and wake them up. What they didn't know was that this would happen before they reached Stage 2 sleep, while they were still in the sleep period when the imagination finds associations between seemingly dissimilar ideas that can lead to creative solutions to problems. The peculiar five-minute wonder of Stage 1 sleep has no known scientific benefits, but so much lore surrounds it that I'm going to take off my lab coat for a moment and delve into the mysterious realm known as the hypnogogic nap.

Hypnogogia, a term coined by 19th-century French psychologist Alfred Maury, refers to the hallucinatory state called sleep-onset dreaming that people enter into when falling asleep, a time that is not fully divorced from waking consciousness. In this state, dreamlike thoughts begin to mix with ideas of the day. The subconscious mind has free reign, which is why it's often used as a tool by lucid dreamers, creative thinkers and mystic seekers, many of whom swear they can will themselves to maintain this state longer than nature's allotted five minutes.

Harvard researcher Robert Stickgold studied sleep-onset dreaming by having subjects learn the video game Tetris. He had them train during the day, then woke them up at night just as they reached sleep-onset dreaming and asked them to write down any imagery they remembered. The majority of subjects reported seeing Tetris pieces falling as they played the game in their minds.

During the first few days of your trip, try to schedule a 20-to-30-minute nap in the afternoon. This will discharge some of your sleep debt while giving you a touch of SWS (which will allow you to stay up longer), but, more importantly, it will provide the sustained alertness and energizing benefits of Stage 2 sleep. Then, as your return date approaches, reverse the sleep adjustment schedule and you'll be back to your normal self—and normal schedule—in no time.

But Stickgold took his inquiry further. He used subjects with severe amnesia who could not create memories that would last longer than a minute after the experience. When shown how to play Tetris, these subjects forgot the rules of the game if they turned even momentarily away from the screen. However, when woken up and asked what they'd been dreaming about, they reported imagery like interestingly shaped tiles falling from the sky into a garden where they had to fit them together. This shows that the reviewing of previous experiences during sleep occurs even in people who cannot consciously form memories.

The value of the information we review in our hypnogogic naps—and what function it serves in our overall experience—has yet to be studied. But we have the following evidence from the 19th-century German chemist Friedrich August Kekulé, who wrote after months of frustrating investigation into the structure of the benzene molecule:

> I turned my chair toward the fireplace and sank into a doze. Again the atoms were flitting before my eyes. Smaller groups now kept modestly in the background. My mind's eye, sharpened by repeated visions of a similar sort, now distinguished larger structures of varying forms. Long rows frequently rose together, all in movement, winding and turning like serpents; and see! what was that? One of the serpents seized its own tail and the form whirled mockingly before my eyes. I came awake like a flash of lightning.

The vision of the mythical serpent known as the Uroboros led Kekulé to realize that the atoms did not form a chain at all, but instead that the ends met in a closed circle. His discovery of the benzene ring laid the foundation for the entire science of organic chemistry. To his fellow scientists Kekulé exhorted: "Let us learn to dream!"

If you're arriving at night, remember to consider the danger zones that can interfere with your nocturnal sleep. Be sure to keep yourself awake at least two hours before your intended bedtime. On planes, this tends not to be a problem. Once you factor in the 20 minutes or so before landing when you have to "bring your seat forward and return your tray table to its upright and locked position," plus the time necessary to retrieve your luggage and get to your final destination, you're pretty much within the two-hour safety buffer. Remember, anything less than two to three hours between waking up from a nap and going to sleep for the night will put you in danger of stealing from your core nocturnal sleep needs. If you're on a short flight, consider the rules of Optimized Napping so you can avoid sleep inertia. Restrict yourself to a light 20-minute nap, but on longer flights feel free to luxuriate in a full-cycle nap (90 minutes or more of sleep). Indeed, NASA research studies advise airline pilots to take one 40-minute nap for every nine hours of flying time. Put this cutting-edge research to work for you.

CHAPTER 10

A nap-positive society

I n the annals of great nappers, 42-year-old Anne-Marie McDermott is a virtuoso. Literally. When she was 12 years old, she performed Mendelssohn's Concerto in G minor with a full orchestra at Carnegie Hall. By her mid-teens, her schedule was so hectic that her mentor at the Manhattan School of Music suggested meditation, but she discovered napping instead.

Since then, Anne-Marie has performed around the world with such illustrious companies as the New York Philharmonic, Moscow Virtuosi and the Brandenburg Ensemble. By age 22, napping had become as integral a part of her routine as practicing scales. "I treat it almost like a religious thing," she says. "My nap on concert days is the most critical of all, since I have to be at my optimal level of performance when I take the stage." Rising at 9 A.M., she goes to the hall and rehearses the evening's program from 10 to 1 P.M. "in a supernonemotional way—cold, clinical and slow." Then she returns home or to her hotel to take care of business, answering e-mails and so on, before enjoying a nap-friendly lunch, usually a turkey and cheese sandwich. "I base the length of my nap on how much concentration I need that evening," she explains. "Sometimes an hour is enough, but if it's a high-pressure concert—if I'm the soloist carrying the entire performance, for instance—I'll need something longer, maybe an hour and a half to two hours. But I always wake up two and a half hours before the concert to take a shower and put on my makeup."

Anne-Marie reports that she never feels fuzzy after her nap, because of the pre-performance adrenaline, the shower and saving her coffee fix for after her nap. She also tries to maintain the same schedule on nonconcert days, and when events conspire to take away any opportunity for a long nap, she still lays her head down on her dressing table before the show and "zones out" for 10 minutes.

If ever a real live napper inhabited that "perfect world" we imagined in Chapter 1, it is this musical prodigy. Thanks to her specialized skills and the leeway afforded by our society to recognized "creative types," Anne-Marie is allowed the time, space and permission to nap, and she makes the most of it. A 90-to-120-minute nap is getting her all the benefits we've learned about, including Stage 2 motor enhancement of her agile pianist hands, SWS restoration and clearing of sleep pressure to allow her to have a clear mind and an extended period of productive wake time, and, of course, a healthy shot of REM to keep her creativity high and let her add the emotive touches to the pieces that she so mechanically practiced earlier. She also wakes up either in REM or Stage 2, leaving minimal sleep inertia and allowing her to transition to her evening performance with alertness and calm. Indeed, she says, napping is so common in her profession that the sound you're most likely to hear the afternoon before an evening performance by any given philharmonic orchestra is a symphony of napping musicians!

But what about the rest of us? The people who teach school, raise children, drive trucks, write software, balance corporate accounts or do scientific research? Aren't we entitled to the nap's benefits so we, too, can give our best performance?

In a perfect world, society would grant all of us the space to become virtuoso nappers. And getting there from here is the final step in the napper's journey. It's one we must all take together—with science at our side—if we are to succeed.

Workers of the world, nap!

If you've gotten this far, you're one of us: a napper. Welcome. And congratulations. You have taken an important step in redesigning your life to be healthier, happier and younger-looking, not to mention, safer, smarter and more productive. Who could have guessed a little nap could do all that? For some of you, this book might have encouraged you to take your first nap. Longtime nappers will have gained a new appreciation of a beloved, albeit little understood aspect of their lives and learned a few new tips on how to use their naps more effectively. Now it's time for nappers to not only stand up and be counted, but also to get proactive. You need only share what you've learned here and of course lead by example to find your friends and family joining you on the nap bandwagon. Creating a nap-friendly workplace is another matter.

No one knows this better than author and clinical psychologist Bill Anthony. A third-generation napper, he and his wife, Camille, instilled in their family a healthy appreciation for napping. With grandchildren of their own, the Anthonys have now perpetuated the tradition into the fifth generation. "In our household," says Bill, "if someone wants to curl up for a snooze, the rest of the family honors that person's wish by being quiet and staying out of the way." The Anthonys have pooled their ideas into two delightful books on napping (*The Art of Napping* and *The Art of Napping at Work*). More importantly, they have been instrumental in instituting National Napping Day, celebrated the first Monday after daylight saving time starts, and their tireless lobbying in person, in print and on TV has helped businesses, particularly in the United States, wake up to the benefits of going to sleep.

While universal napping might sound like an impossible (midday) dream, there are encouraging signs that the anti-nap trend set in motion with the first mechanical timepieces has begun to reverse. Surprisingly, this is occurring most dramatically in the

119

more industrialized nations of northern Europe, which were the first to jettison the practice in their pell-mell rush to industrialize. A recent study of napping behavior in Europe found that Germany leads the continent with 22 percent of the working population napping at least three times a week. (By German law, the hours between 1 and 3 P.M., Monday through Saturday, are reserved for the *Mittagsruhe,* or midday rest, and no loud or unusual noises are permitted which would disturb people who may be napping). The U.K. runs a distant second, while the traditional siesta countries of Italy and Spain trail far behind.

On a recent visit to my birthplace, Denmark, I discovered that the town of Hillerød, a provincial municipality of around 37,000 people located 20 miles northwest of Copenhagen, has a workplace napping policy in effect for all its civil servants. This "power napping experiment," as it was called, occurred because back in 2002 Mayor Nick Haekkerup got a call from a magazine reporter asking him why he didn't let his 3,500 municipal employees nap. The reporter cited much of the same research you are now familiar with, demonstrating that napping is not only helpful in staving off fatigue but also has many emotional and cognitive benefits. A similar program had already been tried with great success in Vechta, Germany, whose city manager was inspired by a power napping presentation he attended in the United States.

Mayor Haekkerup was already in the midst of studying ways to improve the wellness of his employees, but the idea of a napping policy hadn't occurred to him even though he'd been a devoted napper since his days as a Ph.D. student at the University of Copenhagen. He circulated a questionnaire asking the civil servants how much sleep they got, how tired they were during the day, how much their work and happiness was affected by sleepiness and whether they liked to nap at work. The employees responded with a resounding yawn on the fatigue poll and a big YES on the napping question. ScanSleep, a Danish sleep clinic, joined the project and helped to plan a six-week trial study—much like our six-week program—to determine what effect instituting napping in the workplace would have. They found (no surprise) that when workers are allowed to nap, they feel less tired, work better and report greater job satisfaction. Haekkerup decided that it should be part of workplace policy, although he left it up to each individual business how to work it out. "People laughed when they first heard about it," he says, "but the program is over two years old and not only is it thriving, but other institutions in Denmark—hospitals, transportation departments and oil industries—have now adopted it."

Thanks to the efforts of the Anthonys and others, businesses in the United States have also begun to see the wisdom of workplace napping. Nike's employees "do it," and the Connecticut company Yarde Metals actively encourages it by providing a nap area for employees. Burlington Northern Santa Fe Railroad allows train conductors and engineers to take naps of up to 45 minutes in length. Another 24-hour operation, Nova Chemicals, built rooms where its production workers can nap, and Deloitte Consulting did the same for its nine-to-fivers. (At another consulting company, 42, employees have to book the nap room in advance because demand has outstripped the supply of couch space!)

But nowhere is the napping trend more entrenched than in the progressive business environment of Silicon Valley, where new ideas are more likely to be embraced than feared. One of the local pioneers was TRC Lowney Associates, a geotechnical and environmental engineering firm located in Mountain View, where on-site napping has been the rule since the company's inception in 1969. The forward-thinking founder, John Lowney, believed it was good business to reduce stress on the job and promote a healthy workplace culture. He put pictures on the walls and plants all through the office and, best of all, turned an extra room into a "quiet room," complete with a large, nap-friendly couch. "There's no stigma against napping here," says Barry Butler, a staff engineer and one of the 45 people at the office who make regular trips to the room. "As long as employees complete their work and do so professionally, they're free to do whatever they need to do."

But the modern workplace still has a long way to go. In 2000, the National Sleep Foundation polled U.S. workers and found that more than 80 percent of them said their employers didn't allow naps, while Cornell University professor James Maas (author of the bestseller *Power Sleep*) estimates that these days around 40 percent do it on the sly anyway.

Power points of workplace napping

So how do you get your employer to see the wisdom of allowing you to nap at work? The key to getting the go-ahead is a compelling proposal that looks at the arrangement through the employer's eyes. What risks does it present to the organization? What might the benefits be? And why might this organization be especially suitable or unsuitable for workplace napping?

Remember that your employer's priority is the operation of the business, not your personal life. If you say things like "I want to nap at work because I have insomnia," not only do you fail to strike the proper professional tone, but you present yourself as a liability as opposed to someone who has an innovative idea to create a more efficient workplace. Company managers are worried about meeting deadlines, productivity and actual work being completed. So when you approach your supervisor, be sure your presentation speaks to those concerns.

This means you have to communicate how it benefits *them* to invest in a nap room so they don't only picture people sleeping who would otherwise be at their desks answering phones or working on projects. Fortunately for you, these points are easy to make.

Benefit #1: Napping reduces absenteeism.
A 1999 study concluded that healthy employees often miss work because of fatigue and fatigue-related illness. Sleep deprivation has been shown to weaken the immune system, contribute to depression and lower motivation, alertness and cognition. Napping leads to an increase in the health and well-being of your employees and thus reduces days off.

Benefit #2: Napping increases productivity.
NASA napping studies report an average productivity increase of 13 percent. Other studies show equally positive results for alertness, memory processing and decision-making.

Benefit #3: Napping increases employee retention.
A key concept of napping is the ability to better balance work/personal life with health needs. It's an option more and more employees are demanding. A napping arrangement allows the organization to increase employee satisfaction, morale and productivity.

Benefit #4: Napping saves money. Lots of it.
Compare a nap room with the cost of building a gym, hiring a massage therapist or bringing on wellness trainers, and the nap comes out looking like a bargain.

Now that you've addressed your employer's concerns, you're well on your way to crafting a convincing proposal. To make your case, start by briefly reviewing the reasons you want to build a nap environment. Concentrate on quality-of-life issues and productivity. Stress the character traits, skills and accomplishments that make your office the perfect candidate for a power napping culture.

Next, address the logistics. Explain where a nap room could be constructed. What would be needed: a comfy easy chair or couch, a side table with a soft bulb lamp and a blanket. Outline the equipment you already have and anything else you may need to create the space with the least amount of trouble. Explain that any costs will be more than offset by the savings. How many people will use it? At what time? How will it be organized so that there will be an equal napping opportunity for everyone? Find a community of nappers or would-be nappers and band together. Try to quantify how much fatigue decreases what you and your coworkers are able to accomplish in a day, a week or a year. Offer your employer a list of reasonable goals that can be used to evaluate the success of the napping arrangement.

Finally, if your boss still isn't comfortable with the idea, suggest a six-week to three-month trial. You can even suggest conducting the kind of study the mayor of Hillerød used—the six-week one that you did on yourself. Offer to distribute the program to willing participants yourself. Then begin a two-week nap training period using the scientifically proven relaxation methods in this book to help new nappers fall asleep. And then take the sleep health assessment again for two more weeks. Your results will be a powerful tool in creating a solid factual argument for napping in your workplace and an example for other businesses and organizations to follow.

This way, you will create a more perfect world not just for yourself but for everybody else to enjoy.

Appendix

Glossary

Actigraphy: A method used to study sleep/wake patterns and circadian rhythms by assessing movement, most commonly of the wrist.

Adenosine: A nucleoside that plays an important role in triggering the urge to sleep. Stimulants, such as caffeine in coffee, often bind to adenosine receptors, thereby blocking the drowsiness trigger.

Alpha wave: A pattern of smooth, regular electrical oscillations in the human brain that occurs when an individual is awake and relaxed. Alpha waves have a recorded frequency of 8 to 13 hertz.

Amphetamine: A colorless, volatile liquid, $C_9H_{13}N$, used as a central nervous system stimulant in the treatment of certain conditions, such as attention deficit hyperactivity disorder, depression and narcolepsy; often abused illegally as a stimulant.

Amplitude: The magnitude of a wave's oscillation.

Anabolic hormone: A class of hormones that promote cell growth and division, resulting in growth of several types of tissues, particularly muscle and bone.

Beta wave: The second most common waveform occurring in the adult brain, characteristically having a frequency of 13 to 30 cycles per second. It is associated with an alert waking state but can also indicate anxiety or apprehension.

Biological clock: See *Circadian rhythm.*

Biphasic sleep: Sleep that occurs in two periods during the 24-hour period.

Brain wave: A rhythmic fluctuation of electric potential between parts of the brain, as seen in an electroencephalogram.

Caffeine: A bitter alkaloid, $C_8H_{10}N_4O_2$, found especially in coffee, tea and cola nuts and used medicinally as a stimulant and/or diuretic. Also known as trimethylxanthine.

Catabolic hormone: A hormone that promotes the metabolic breakdown of complex molecules into simpler ones, often resulting in a release of energy.

Central nervous system: The part of the nervous system to which sensory impulses are transmitted and from which motor impulses pass out, and which supervises and coordinates the activity of the entire nervous system. In vertebrates, this consists of the brain and spinal cord.

Circadian rhythm: An activity cycle based on the 24-hour day; exhibited by humans and most other organisms. The innate rhythm of behavior and body activity in living things is called the biological clock.

Cognitive nap aversion: An inability to nap due to negative information or beliefs about napping.

Compensatory napping: Napping after sleep deprivation has already occurred.

Coping strategy: An adaptive behavior to an extreme circumstance.

Core sleep: The minimum amount of sleep considered necessary to maintain essential brain processes, often cited as 5.5 hours in the case of humans.

Cortisol: An adrenal cortex hormone that takes part in carbohydrate and protein metabolism.

Delta wave: A slow brain wave, having a frequency of fewer than six cycles per second, emanating from the forward portion of the brain; associated with slow-wave sleep in normal adults.

Depression: 1) A psychiatric disorder characterized by an inability to concentrate, insomnia, loss of appetite, anhedonia, feelings of extreme sadness, guilt, helplessness and hopelessness, and thoughts of death; 2) a reduction in physiological vigor or activity.

Designer nap: See *Optimized Napping*.

Dexedrine: Trade name for dextroamphetamine.

Electroencephalogram (EEG): The tracing of brain waves recorded by electrodes placed on the scalp.

Emotional memory: Refers to both the enhancement of memory processing due to emotional value and the association of emotional value to an object or experience due to the presence of an emotionally active stimulus.

Excessive daytime sleepiness (EDS): Subjective report of difficulty in staying awake, accompanied by a ready entrance into sleep when the individual is sedentary.

Fatigue: Tiredness due to lack of sleep and/or overexertion.

Fatigue Denial: Being cognitively blind to one's own state of fatigue; usually results in overestimating one's level of ability.

Frequency: The number of times an event occurs per unit of time.

Functional magnetic resonance imaging (fMRI): An imaging technique that relies on the magnetic signals detected in an activated brain region in relation to its degree of oxygenation, i.e., blood flow.

Geniculate nuclei: A component of the thalamus that relays auditory and visual information from the sense organs to the brain.

Growth hormone: A polypeptide hormone secreted by the anterior lobe of the pituitary gland that promotes growth and repair of body tissue.

Homeostatic drive: The body's constant effort to maintain homeostasis or equilibrium.

Hypnogogic nap/hypnogogic state: An intermediate state between consciousness and sleep, thought by many to allow for greater creativity and even mystical apprehension.

Hypomanic state: A state of mind or behavior that is "below" mania, often brought on by sleep deprivation. An individual in this state typically exhibits euphoria, overactivity, disinhibition, impulsivity, a decreased need for sleep and/or hypersexuality, but not in such a pronounced fashion as to be considered clinically manic.

Jet lag: A temporary disruption of normal circadian rhythm as a result of high-speed travel across several time zones, typically in a jet aircraft, causing fatigue and varied constitutional symptoms.

"K" complexes: Sharp, negative, high-voltage EEG waves, followed by slower, positive components, whose spontaneous appearances characterize Stage 2 sleep, although they also appear during slow-wave sleep (SWS). "K" complexes can be elicited during sleep by external (particularly auditory) stimuli as well. See also *Sleep spindles*.

Lark: An individual whose high-functioning hours occur during the early morning; can be a symptom of advanced sleep phase.

Leptin: A peptide hormone produced by fat cells that plays a role in body weight regulation by suppressing appetite and burning fat stored in adipose tissue.

Long-term depression (LTD): The weakening of neuronal synapses that occurs during slow-wave sleep and is evident in the delta wave; important for clearing of old memory traces and motor learning.

Long-term potentiation (LTP): A long-lasting strengthening of the response of a nerve cell to stimulation; thought to be related to learning and long-term memory.

Lucid dreaming: Consciously perceiving and recognizing that one is in a dream during sleep, sometimes leading to control over the "dreamscape," i.e., the world within the dream.

Maggie's Law: First U.S. law (passed in New Jersey) specifically stating that a sleep-deprived driver is a reckless driver who can therefore be convicted of vehicular homicide.

Melatonin: A hormone derived from serotonin and produced by the pineal gland; plays a role in sleep, aging and reproduction in mammals.

Memory consolidation: The process of storing information for long-term retention.

Microsleep: A period of sleep that lasts up to a few seconds, usually experienced by people who suffer from narcolepsy or sleep deprivation.

Modafinil: An FDA-approved stimulant used to counteract excessive sleepiness. It works by changing the amounts of certain natural substances in the area of the brain that controls sleep and wakefulness. Trade name: Provigil.

Monophasic sleep: Sleep that occurs in only one period per day.

Motor learning: Refers to a set of internal processes associated with practice or experience leading to long-term increases in accuracy and speed of motor responses.

Multiphasic sleep: See *Polyphasic sleep.*

Nap blocker: Anything that prevents the ability to nap.

Nap nod: An awkward head motion caused by falling asleep in a position where the head is not supported.

Napping clubs: Social groups formed on the basis of a common love of napping.

Narcolepsy: A disorder characterized by sudden and uncontrollable, though often brief, attacks of deep sleep, sometimes accompanied by paralysis and hallucinations.

National Napping Day: The first Monday after the beginning of daylight saving time; designed to heighten awareness of the health and productivity benefits of napping.

Neuromotor: Relating to a nerve fiber or impulse that controls or affects motor activity.

Neuron: Any of the impulse-conducting cells that constitute the brain, spinal cord and nerves.

Neurotransmitter: A chemical substance released from one neuron that transmits a signal to the next neuron.

Noise canceler: A device that matches the sound waves in an environment with equal amplitude and opposite phase, causing the sensory experience of noise to be canceled out.

Occipital cortex: The part of the brain responsible for visual processing.

Operational maintenance nap: A nap taken during work but before serious sleepiness and fatigue has set in.

Operational napping: Napping during work hours.

Operational recovery nap: A nap taken after a period of sleep deprivation with the aim of restoring some alertness.

Optimized Napping: A scientific method used for calculating the exact time and length of a nap to achieve the desired proportion of sleep stages based on an individual's unique set of needs, i.e., a designer nap.

Owl: An individual whose high-functioning hours occur at night; can be a symptom of delayed sleep phase.

Paradoxical sleep: See *Rapid eye movement (REM)*.

PGO waves: Spiky waves that indicate the onset of rapid eye movement (REM) sleep, so named because of the sites in the brain where they can be easily recorded: the pons (where they originate), the lateral geniculate nucleus and the occipital (visual) cortex.

Photosensitivity: Sensitivity or responsiveness to light.

Polyphasic sleep: Sleep that occurs in multiple periods throughout the day.

Polyphasic ultrashort sleep: A practice developed by Claudio Stampi intended to reduce sleep time to 2 to 5 hours daily. This is achieved by spreading out sleep into short naps of 20 to 45 minutes throughout the day. Also known as Überman napping.

Polysomnography: The technique or process of using a polygraph to make a continuous record during sleep of multiple physiological variables (e.g., breathing, heart rate and muscle activity) through the use of electrodes.

Pons: The part of the brain stem that relays sensory information between the cerebellum and cerebrum; part of the trigger for rapid eye movement (REM) sleep.

Positron-emission tomography (PET): A technology that creates a cross-sectional image of metabolic activity (often in the brain) by injecting a slightly radioactive solution into the bloodstream and mapping the sites where these molecules are absorbed.

Post-lunch dip: A feeling of tiredness that occurs in the early afternoon. Erroneously thought to be caused by the digestion process following lunch, this phenomenon occurs whether or not a meal has been consumed.

Potentiation: The process whereby a biochemical or physiological action or effect is promoted or strengthened.

Power nap: A short nap (20 minutes or less) composed almost completely of Stage 2 sleep (also called Stage 2 nap). The term was first coined by sleep researcher James B. Maas.

Prefrontal cortex: The region of the frontal lobe involved in cognitive behavior and motor planning.

Preventive nap: A nap taken prior to an operational episode.

Prophylactic napping: Napping in anticipation of a period when sleep will not be possible.

Provigil: See *Modafinil.*

Rapid eye movement (REM): A stage in the normal sleep cycle during which vivid dreams occur and the body undergoes marked changes including rapid eye movement, muscle atonia and increased pulse rate and brain activity; characterized by fast, low-voltage activity and sawtooth waves. Once called "paradoxical sleep" due to the brain's electrical similarity to the waking state.

Serotonin: A neurotransmitter known to play an important role in mood, sleep, emesis (vomiting), sexuality and appetite; may facilitate the onset of sleep by dampening the individual's response to sensory input.

Shadow cycles: The unmanifested continuation of REM and slow-wave sleep (SWS) cycles during wakefulness; allow naps to vary in their sleep quality depending on what time these cycles are "accessed."

Siesta: A tradition of sleeping in the afternoon, typically occurring in Mediterranean regions; usually follows a big lunch and involves closing shops till late afternoon.

Sleep cycle: A period of sleep in which the brain passes through all five sleep stages. This cycle of approximately 90 minutes is repeated four to six times each night.

Sleep debt: A term characterizing the cumulative effects of sleep deprivation.

Sleep deprivation: A condition that results from lack of adequate sleep.

Sleep inertia: A feeling of grogginess and/or sleepiness that occurs after waking up from slow-wave sleep (SWS).

Sleep interference: Interruption of sleep resulting in arousal and wakefulness.

Sleep-onset dreaming: Images and experiences that occur during the moments following the transition from the waking state to sleep.

Sleep pressure: The characterization of the biological need for sleep at any given moment.

Sleep spindles: Episodically appearing spindle-shaped aggregates of 12 to 14 hertz with a duration of 0.5 to 1.5 seconds; one of the identifying EEG features of Stage 2 sleep. See also *"K" complexes.*

Sleep stage: One of five differentiated periods of sleep (Stage 1, Stage 2, Stage 3, Stage 4, REM), each characterized by its own electrical signature.

Slow-wave sleep (SWS): Stage 3 and Stage 4 of the sleep cycle; the deepest stage of sleep.

Spatial orientation: The process of aligning or positioning oneself or an object in a three-dimensional space with respect to a specific direction or reference system; relies on REM sleep for solid establishment.

Spindles: See *Sleep spindles.*

Stage 1 sleep: A transition stage of sleep occurring between the waking state and Stage 2 sleep. Stage 1 normally assumes 2 to 5 percent of total sleep.

Stage 2 nap: See *Power nap.*

Stage 2 sleep: A sleep stage characterized by sleep spindles and "K" complexes against a relatively low-voltage, mixed-frequency EEG background.

Stage 3 sleep: A deep-sleep stage defined by 20 to 50 percent of the period (30-second epoch), consisting of EEG waves of less than 2 hertz; with Stage 4, constitutes slow-wave sleep (SWS).

Stage 4 sleep: Identical to Stage 3 except that slow, high-voltage EEG waves exceed 50 percent of the period; with Stage 3, constitutes slow-wave sleep (SWS).

Stimulant: An agent, typically a chemical such as caffeine, that temporarily arouses or accelerates physiological or organic activity;

can be used to counteract sleepiness.

String galvanometer: An early device that used thin filament fibers to detect tiny oscillating currents, such as those given off by the brain and heart. This procedure led to the utilization of the electroencephalogram (EEG) and electrocardiogram (ECG) in modern science.

Sugar high: Hyperactivity brought on by eating a lot of sugar.

Thalamus: An ovoid mass of neurons located deep within the forebrain that relays sensory information to and from the cerebral cortex.

Theta wave: A waveform on an electroencephalogram typified by a frequency of 4 to 8 hertz; typically found in Stage 1 and REM sleep.

Thyroid gland: An endocrine gland located in front of and on either side of the trachea in humans; responsible for regulating metabolic rate.

Trimethylxanthine: See *Caffeine*.

Tryptophan: An essential amino acid, $C_{11}H_{12}N_2O_2$, formed from proteins during digestion of certain foods; believed to bring on drowsiness.

Type A Fallacy: The (erroneous) argument that working more hours at the expense of adequate sleep will yield higher productivity.

Überman napping: See *Polyphasic ultrashort sleep.*

Ultimate nap: A nap with equal amounts of slow-wave sleep and REM sleep.

Visual learning: A type of learning in which the individual sharpens or otherwise improves his or her ability to detect and discriminate visual targets.

Vivid dreaming: The surreal narrative episodes that occur during REM sleep; what people generally think of when they mention dreams.

Waking after sleep onset (WASO): Any period spent awake after initial sleep onset but before final awakening.

The Scientific Formula for Creating the Precise Nap to Suit Your Needs

Although most people will be content with the level of complexity described in Chapter 6, I've included the Optimized Napping formula and a brief explanation for those readers interested in working a little more precision into their napping habits.

Nap science's own theory of relativity expresses the relationship between the stages of sleep that are contained in any given nap. If N stands for the quality of your nap, R for the circadian effect on REM, S for sleep pressure and the numeral 2 for Stage 2, we can express the nap formula as:

$$N = R/S+2$$

Using the formula, which is really a summation of our knowledge of Stage 2, slow-wave sleep (SWS) and REM sleep, we can better estimate the quality of any given nap. Let's start with Stage 2, the constant in our equation. The transitional element between all the major phases of sleep, it also serves as your entryway into a nice long nap, which is why we know that the first 20 minutes of your nap will be Stage 2. After that period, you will travel deeper into slow-wave sleep, then back up to Stage 2, then over to REM, then around again to Stage 2. This means that for naps that are longer than 20 minutes, you can calculate that Stage 2 will constitute 60 percent of the full 90-minute cycle.

That's pretty simple. But to complicate matters, let's examine the relationship between SWS and REM, which makes up the rest of a 90-minute nap, or 40 percent. We know that SWS must precede REM within each cycle since the body's need for SWS must be satiated before REM is allowed to do its work. This means that REM and SWS have a kind of antagonistic relationship. When SWS is high, REM is low, and when REM is holding court, SWS is shunted to the margins. This is why we express this part of the equation as R/S. We're not dividing anything here, just expressing the inverse relationship between the two values. So within the first few hours after you've woken up, your sleep pressure is low and thus the denominator (S) will be small, allowing the numerator (R) to suck up the majority of the 40 percent. But as your hours awake increase, sleep pressure will increase and with it the denominator (S). This means that REM sleep will have to start sharing more of the 40 percent since each hour later will see more SWS crowding into the nap.

Knowing how all these stages interact will prepare you to manipulate them to create your own personalized nap—or at least to understand what benefits you've received from the nap you've just taken.

For a more interactive version of the formula, in which you can enter in your own specific nap variables, visit my Web site: saramednick.com.

About the Authors

Sara Mednick, a research scientist at the Salk Institute for Biological Studies in La Jolla, California, received her Ph.D. in psychology from Harvard University. The leading expert in the field of napping research, she has worked with numerous academic institutions, the military, and private businesses. Her napping research has been covered by CNN, Reuters TV, NPR, *The Economist, The Wall Street Journal, Consumer Reports, Health Journal, Reader's Digest, The New York Times, Real Simple, Time* and *Men's Journal.*

Mark Ehrman is a freelance writer living in Los Angeles. His work regularly appears in the *Los Angeles Times, Playboy, InStyle,* and many other papers and magazines.